Clinical Simulations
in Laboratory Medicine

SHAUNA C. ANDERSON
PhD, CLS(NCA), MT(ASCP)C
Program Director, Clinical Laboratory Science
Associate Professor, Department of Microbiology
Brigham Young University
Provo, Utah

JOYCE A. BEHRENS
MS, CLS(NCA), MT(ASCP)
Assistant Professor, Department of Laboratory Medicine
University of Washington
Seattle, Washington

SUSAN COCKAYNE
MS, CLS(NCA), MT(ASCP)
Instructor, Department of Microbiology
Brigham Young University
Provo, Utah

CAROL N. LECRONE
MS, CLS(NCA), MT(ASCP)
Program Director, Medical Technology
Assistant Professor, Department of Laboratory Medicine
University of Washington
Seattle, Washington

KEILA B. POULSEN
BS, CLS(NCA)H, MT(ASCP)H,SH
Hematology Supervisor
Eastern Idaho Regional Medical Center
Idaho Falls, Idaho

Clinical Simulations in Laboratory Medicine

J. B. Lippincott Company

PHILADELPHIA · LONDON · MEXICO · NEW YORK

SÃO PAULO · SYDNEY

Acquisitions Editor: Lisa Biello
Sponsoring Editor: Sanford Robinson
Manuscript Editor: Linda Fitzpatrick
Design Director: Tracy Baldwin
Design Coordinator: Don Shenkle

Designer: Carl Gross
Production Supervisor: J. Corey Gray
Production Coordinator: Barney Fernandes
Compositor: Bi-Comp, Inc.
Printer/Binder: Martin Printing Co.

ISBN 0-397-50746-1

6 5 4 3 2 1

The authors and publisher have exerted every effort to ensure that drug selection and dosage set forth in this text are in accord with current recommendations and practice at the time of publication. However, in view of ongoing research, changes in government regulations, and the constant flow of information relating to drug therapy and drug reactions, the reader is urged to check the package insert for each drug for any change in indications and dosage and for added warnings and precautions. This is particularly important when the recommended agent is a new or infrequently employed drug.

Preface

CLINICAL SIMULATIONS IN LABORATORY MEDICINE is designed to assist clinical laboratory scientists, dietitians, respiratory therapists, nurses, physicians, medical students, and other members of the health care team in interpreting, evaluating, and correlating clinical laboratory data with the pathophysiology of disease states. In this book, the written simulation is used as a method of teaching problem-solving skills involving these data. At the beginning of each case, a short scenario provides information that defines a problem. After the problem is established, the reader is asked to respond to questions about the case by gently rubbing the bracketed area beneath the choice with a special marker that is supplied with the book. By selecting a response, the reader receives feedback concerning his choice and further instructions.

Two types of written clinical simulations have been incorporated: linear and branching. The linear type is employed to approach a straightforward problem. The case will proceed from one section to the next and will require the selection of a correct answer or answers. Immediate feedback is provided with a latent-image printing process. The problem continues until all pertinent data relating to the disease state are elucidated.

The branching technique is used to present a more complex problem. This technique is similar to the linear type in that it is composed of a short introduction that establishes a problem but differs in the fact that, as the case develops, two or more paths may be pursued, depending on previous choices rather than proceeding in sequential steps.

Written simulations can also provide relevant information in health-related problems without actual patient contact. This instructional technique should be implemented in the later stages of the curriculum, when the background knowledge has already been taught.

The authors hope that the reader will find that this book provides a unique and exciting instructional technique and a rewarding learning experience.

Shauna C. Anderson, PhD, CLS, MT

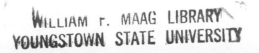

Acknowledgments

APPRECIATION IS EXTENDED to our families and Brigham Young University for their support and to the laboratory personnel at Columbus Hospital, Great Falls, Montana for providing data. Special thanks are given to Sarah C. Dawson for proofreading and critiquing the material and to Stephanie George for the preparation of the manuscript.

SCA and SC

SPECIAL ACKNOWLEDGMENT IS GIVEN to Dr. Wayne Chandler of the Department of Laboratory Medicine, University of Washington, and to Dr. Richard Counts of the Puget Sound Blood Center for assistance in providing appropriate material for these case studies. My appreciation is also extended to Dr. Chandler for his willingness to critique the cases.

JAB

SPECIAL ACKNOWLEDGMENT IS GIVEN to the technologists in the Hemolysis Laboratory, University Hospital, and to Roberta Foster-Smith, Group Health, for assistance in providing appropriate case data for this publication. My appreciation is also extended to Dr. James C. Detter for his willingness to critique the cases.

CNL

APPRECIATION IS EXTENDED to my family for their patience and support and to the Hematology Staff at Eastern Idaho Regional Medical Center for their assistance in critiquing the cases. My appreciation is also given to Linda Barna for her efforts in providing data and extensive critiquing of this material and to Shauna Anderson for her assistance and this opportunity.

KBP

Contents

Case 1

A 39-YEAR-OLD WOMAN presents to her physician with heat intolerance and heart palpitations. She also complains of excessive lacrimation and a sandy sensation in her eyes. She has been under a physician's care and is currently taking Dilantin. On physical examination her pulse is 125/minute; her blood pressure is 135/70; and her skin is warm and moist. The following laboratory tests were performed:

Total T_4 (TT$_4$) = 14.2 μg/dl (4.5–13.0)
Resin T_3 Uptake (RT$_3$U) = 40% (25–35)

Which of the following laboratory determinations would be of value in determining whether the Dilantin therapy was interfering with the results? (Select one.)

1. Serum T_3 (T$_3$)
   [   ]
2. Free T_4 index (FT$_4$I)
   [   ]
3. Thyroid-stimulating hormone (TSH) level
   [   ]
4. Thyroxine-binding globulin (TBG) level
   [   ]

Section A
The FT$_4$I is calculated from the following formula:

$$FT_4I = TT_4 \times RT_3U \text{ ratio}$$
$$TT_4 = 14.2 \ \mu g/dl$$
$$RT_3U = 40\% \ (normal = 30\%)$$
$$RT_3U \text{ ratio} = 40/30 = 1.33$$

$$FT_4I = 14.2 \times 1.33 = 18.9 \ (4.5–13.0)$$

If the increased RT_3U were due to Dilantin therapy alone, the TT_4 value would be decreased, and when the TT_4 is calculated, it would be normal.

Go to Section C.

Section B
The increase in the RT_3U during Dilantin therapy is not due to an increase in TBG. Therefore, the TBG would be normal. The increase in the RT_3U is due to a competition mechanism where the Dilantin competes with the thyroid hormones for the binding sites on the TBG.

Go to Section C.

Section C
In order to pinpoint the cause of the hyperthyroidism, which of the following tests would be most beneficial? (Select one.)

1. Serum T_3 (T_3)

   [   ]

2. TSH levels

   [   ]

3. Radioactive iodine uptake (RAIU)

   [   ]

4. T_3 suppression test

   [   ]

5. Thyroid antibodies

   [   ]

Section D
Serum T_3 is measured by radioimmunoassay techniques. It has a high discriminant value in the diagnosis of hyperthyroidism. It is of most value in patients who have symptoms of hyperthyroidism and when the TT_4 is still normal.

Go back to Section C and select another alternative.

Section E
If the hyperthyroidism was caused by a pituitary tumor, the TSH would be elevated. The TSH level on this patient was 5.0 $\mu U/ml$ (5–10).

Go back to Section C and select another alternative.

Section F
In most cases, the RAIU is increased in hyperthyroidism but is not usually needed in making the diagnosis. It has been suggested that the primary use of the test is in differentiating the causes of hyperthyroidism.

Causes of Hyperthyroidism
RAIU is diminished (<5%)
 Recent ingestion of thyroid hormones or iodine
 Thyrotoxicosis factitia
 Thyroiditis (subacute and chronic)
 Struma ovarii
 Metastatic thyroid carcinoma
RAIU is normal or elevated
 Pituitary tumor
 Trophoblastic tumor
 Toxic nodular goiter
 Graves' disease
 Chronic thyroiditis (Hashimoto's disease)

Go back to Section C and select another alternative.

Section G
The thyroid releasing hormone (TRH) stimulation test has replaced the T_3 suppression test because it is both simpler and better tolerated by the patient.

Go back to Section C and select another alternative.

Section H
Which of the following thyroid antibodies would help pinpoint the cause of this patient's hyperthyroidism? (Select one.)
 1. Thyroglobulin antibodies
  [   ]
 2. Thyroid-stimulating immunoglobulins (TSI)
  [   ]
 3. Microsomal antibodies
  [   ]
 4. Colloid antibodies (CA-2)
  [   ]

Section I
Thyroglobulin antibodies can be positive in Hashimoto's disease, Graves' disease, thyroid cancer, and subacute thyroiditis.

Go back to Section H and select another alternative.

Section J
Thyroid-stimulating immunoglobulins are a variety of 7S gamma globulins. They are antibodies to the TSH receptor on the follicular cell of the thyroid. These antibodies have been given many names, including long-acting thyroid stimulator (LATS), LATS-protector (LATS-P), TSH-binding

immunoglobulin (TSII), and thyroid stimulation antibodies (TSAb). The TSI on this patient were positive.

Go to Section M.

Section K
Microsomal antibodies can be positive in Hashimoto's disease, primary myxedema, and thyrotoxicosis.

Go to Section H and select another alternative.

Section L
Antibodies to colloid antigen have been found in about 50% of those patients with subacute thyroiditis and in some patients with Hashimoto's disease who demonstrate no other antibodies. CA-2 antibodies were negative in this patient.

Go to Section M.

Section M
From the patient's laboratory data, which of the following is the most likely cause of the hyperthyroidism? (Select one.)

    1. Pituitary tumor
      [   ]

    2. Trophoblastic tumor
      [   ]

    3. Toxic nodular goiter
      [   ]

    4. Graves' disease
      [   ]

    5. Hashimoto's disease
      [   ]

Section N
Hyperthyroidism may occur from TSH secretion as a result of a pituitary adenoma. The TSH will be elevated in spite of an elevated TT_4. The TSH was normal.

Go back to Section M and select another alternative.

Section O
Trophoblastic tumors can cause thyrotoxicosis. These tumors include hydatidiform mole, choriocarcinoma, or embryonal carcinoma of the testis. They secrete human chorionic gonadotropin (HCG). The HCG assay on this patient was negative.

Go back to Section M and select another alternative.

Section P
Toxic multinodular goiter and toxic nodule can cause hyperthyroidism. The structure of the thyroid can be evaluated by the thyroid scan. A multinodular goiter will reveal a patchy uptake of isotope throughout the gland. A single nodule can be classified as "hot," "warm," or "cold," depending on the isotope concentration of the nodule compared to the isotope concentration in surrounding tissue. The thyroid scan in this patient revealed a diffuse uptake.

Go back to Section M and select another alternative.

Section Q
Graves' disease appears to be caused by the production of TSI that interact with the thyroid follicular cell membrane. Therefore, iodine uptake and the synthesis and release of the thyroid hormones are stimulated. This patient has a positive TSI.

Go to Section S.

Section R
About 10% of patients with Hashimoto's disease are chemically hyperthyroid because of excessive secretion of thyroid hormones. These patients may produce TSI and have the same clinical manifestations as those with Graves' disease. In Hashimoto's disease, the RAIU may be elevated or low. If it is elevated, the TT_4 is usually low and the TSH high. If it is low, the TT_4 is usually high and the TSH low. Thyroid biopsy or fine-needle aspiration may differentiate the two disorders. In Hashimoto's disease, there is marked lymphocyte infiltrate with interspersed plasma cells and increased interstitial fibrosis.

Go to Section S.

Section S
What would you expect for each of the following laboratory values?

Creatine Kinase (CK)

1. Elevated
   [   ]
2. Normal
   [   ]
3. Low
   [   ]

Alkaline Phosphatase (ALP)

1. Elevated
   [   ]

2. Normal

[   ]

3. Low

[   ]

Serum Calcium

1. Elevated

[   ]

2. Normal

[   ]

3. Low

[   ]

Cholesterol

1. Elevated

[   ]

2. Normal

[   ]

3. Low

[   ]

Glucose Tolerance Test (GTT)

1. Diabetic curve

[   ]

2. Normal curve

[   ]

3. Hypoglycemic curve

[   ]

White Blood Cell Count

1. Elevated

[   ]

2. Normal

[   ]

3. Low

[   ]

Hematocrit

1. Elevated

[   ]

2. Normal
   [   ]
3. Low
   [   ]

Red Blood Cell Mass

1. Elevated
   [   ]
2. Normal
   [   ]
3. Low
   [   ]

Section T
The CK level is usually half the normal level.

Return to Section S.

Section U
An increased bone turnover causes an elevated ALP. The urinary hydroxy-proline is also elevated.

Return to Section S.

Section V
Thyrotoxicosis results in increased bone turnover, a hypercalciuria, and, in about 10% of patients, a hypercalcemia.

Return to Section S.

Section W
An increased mobilization of fats leads to an increase in free fatty acids, a decrease in serum cholesterol, and a tendency toward ketosis.

Return to Section S.

Section X
Thyroid hormones increase the gastric absorption of glucose and also increase glycogenolysis, thus causing a diabetic curve appearance on the GTT.

Return to Section S.

Section Y
It has been reported that there is a decrease in the white blood cells (WBC) because of a relative decrease in the neutrophils.

Return to Section S.

Section Z

A normocytic, normochromic anemia is commonly seen. The life span of the red blood cell may be moderately shortened with an increased erythroid activity of the marrow; however, with an increased turnover of plasma and red cell iron and an increase in plasma volume, the hematocrit may be normal.

Return to Section S.

Section AA

The red cell mass may be increased due to the excessive demand for oxygen.

Go to the Enrichment Section.

Enrichment Section

Thyrotoxicosis is the name applied to a group of syndromes caused by high levels of thyroid hormones. There are a number of causes of hyperthyroidism, including (1) single or multiple autonomously functioning nodules, (2) thyroiditis, (3) an HCG-secreting tumor, (4) a TSH-secreting pituitary tumor, (5) excessive ingestion of inorganic iodide, (6) thyroid carcinoma, (7) ingestion of excessive exogenous thyroid hormone, and (8) struma ovarii. However, the most common cause of hyperthyroidism is Graves' disease, also known as diffuse toxic goiter.

Graves' disease is thought to be an autoimmune disorder in which several abnormal immunoglobulins are present in the circulation. The trigger mechanism for the excessive production of these antibodies by the B-lymphocytes is unknown. The pathogenesis of the disease appears to be related to the production of TSI, which interact with the TSH receptor to stimulate the uptake of iodide and the synthesis and release of thyroid hormones.

The classic triad of symptoms seen in Graves' disease is diffuse enlargement of the thyroid, ophthalmopathy, and pretibial myxedema. The exophthalmos is due to infiltration of the retro-orbital space with lymphocytes, mast cells, and mucopolysaccharides. In addition to proptosis, ophthalmic symptoms may include increased lacrimation, gritty sensation in the eyes, and diminution in vision. The infiltrative dermopathy is seen in less than 5% of the patients. The skin in the pretibial area of the legs becomes thickened and shiny due to the infiltration with mucopolysaccharides and the chronic inflammation.

The symptoms of thyrotoxicosis are related to the catabolic, hypermetabolic effect, or the increased sensitivity to catecholamines. The increased catabolism in various tissues is responsible for the weight loss, loss of muscle mass, loss of fat stores, exercise intolerance, and easy fatigability. The increased sensitivity to catecholamines is reflected by nervousness, irritability, insomnia, pruritus, tremor, heat intolerance, excessive perspiration, tachycardia, palpitation, and frequent bowel movements.

Bibliography
Blonde L, Riddick FA: Hyperthyroidism: Etiology, diagnosis, and treatment. Hosp Med 16:68–80, 1980
Blonde L, Riddick FA: Hypothyroidism: Clinical features and therapy. Hosp Med 16:52–63, 1980
Hershman JM: Endocrine Pathophysiology: A Patient-Oriented Approach, pp 34–68. Philadelphia, Lea & Febiger, 1982
Mazzaferri EL: Thyrotoxicosis. Postgrad Med 73, No. 4:85–98, 1983
Safrit HF: Diagnosis and management of Graves' disease. Hosp Med 15:74–87, 1979

Case 2

A 65-YEAR-OLD MAN presented with back pain to a hospital clinic. X-rays showed lytic and blastic lesions in his lumbosacral spine. Prostatic examination revealed a nodule in the left lobe. Needle biopsy revealed a poorly differentiated adenocarcinoma.

He was admitted to the hospital for surgery. What preoperative laboratory data would be useful to obtain? (Select as many responses as you feel would be useful.)

1. Hematocrit and hemoglobin
   [   ]

2. White blood cell (WBC)
   [   ]

3. WBC differential
   [   ]

4. Red cell and platelet morphology
   [   ]

5. Prothrombin time (PT), activated partial thromboplastin time (APTT), and thrombin time (TT)
   [   ]

6. Kinetic fibrinogen
   [   ]

7. Platelet count
   [   ]

8. Bleeding time
   [   ]

9. Fibrin split products (fsp)
   [   ]

Section A

What pieces of information would be of concern to you, either in the history or lab data? (Select as many responses as you wish.)

1. Hematocrit and hemoglobin

   [   ]

2. WBC

   [   ]

3. WBC differential

   [   ]

4. Red cell and platelet morphology

   [   ]

5. PT, APTT, TT

   [   ]

6. Kinetic fibrinogen

   [   ]

7. Platelet count

   [   ]

8. Bleeding time

   [   ]

9. fsp

   [   ]

10. Older man with metastatic carcinoma

    [   ]

11. Surgery planned

    [   ]

Section B

At this point in time (prior to surgery), select the most probable diagnosis for this patient, other than carcinoma. (Select one.)

1. Viral infection

   [   ]

2. Acute leukemia

[   ]

3. Acute disseminated intravascular coagulation (DIC)

[   ]

4. Mild chronic DIC

[   ]

5. A hemorrhagic diathesis

[   ]

6. Thrombotic disease

[   ]

Section C

From the following tests, select the test(s) that would be useful and necessary in supporting the diagnosis. (Select as many as necessary.)

1. Fibrinogen survival

[   ]

2. Platelet survival

[   ]

3. Platelet aggregation with adenosine diphosphate (ADP)

[   ]

4. Antithrombin III

[   ]

5. Plasminogen concentration

[   ]

   6. Antiplasmin concentration

[

]

   7. No additional tests needed

[

]

Section D

As part of antihormonal therapy in treating the cancer, a bilateral orchiec-tomy (removal of the testes) was performed the day after admission. Post-operatively the patient was noted to have excessive bleeding from his incision. Which of the following test(s) would be helpful in diagnosis? (Select as many as appropriate.)

   1. PT, APTT, TT

[

]

   2. Kinetic fibrinogen

[   ]

   3. fsp

[   ]

   4. Platelet count

[   ]

   5. Bleeding time

[   ]

   6. Hematocrit and hemoglobin

[

]

   7. WBC

[   ]

Section E

What is the diagnosis for this patient at this time? (Select one.)

   1. Chronic DIC

[   ]

   2. Acute DIC

[

]

Continued

3. Primary fibrinolysis

Section F

The diagnosis of primary fibrinolysis—whether it even actually exists—is controversial. However, if the assumption is made that it does rarely occur, what test(s) would help in differentiating primary fibrinolysis from fibrinolysis secondary to DIC? (Select as many as appropriate.)

1. Paracoagulation test (protamine sulfate or ethanol gelation)

2. Euglobulin clot lysis test (ELT)

3. β-thromboglobulin concentration

4. Antithrombin III (AT III) quantitation

5. Crosslinked D-D dimer fibrin degradation products

Section G

What is the explanation for the partial corrections on these results (PT, APTT, and TT)? (Select one.)

1. Decreased fibrinogen level only

2. Decreased factor VIII:C only

3. Increased concentration of fsp only

4. Combination of decreased coagulation protein(s) and increased fsp

Section H

If a total clottable fibrinogen were done on this patient, what would be the result? (Select one.)

1. The same as the kinetic fibrinogen

2. Higher than the kinetic fibrinogen

Continued

3. Lower than the kinetic fibrinogen

[   ]

Section I

Based on work done by Harker and co-workers, it is possible to predict the bleeding time on a patient with a decreased platelet count between 10 to $100 \times 10^3/\mu l$. Using this, one can then determine if a prolonged bleeding time for a patient with a decreased platelet count is due only to the decrease in platelet number, or if those platelets also show evidence of dysfunction. Using this, the bleeding time on this patient of >30 minutes is which of the following? (Select one.)

1. As predicted

[   ]

2. Shorter than predicted

[   ]

3. Longer than predicted

[   ]

Section J

The bleeding time result is a reflection of which of the following? (Select one.)

1. A decreased platelet count only

[   ]

2. Decreased fibrinogen

[   ]

3. Dysfunctional platelets in addition to decreased number of platelets

$$

$$

Enrichment Section

Disseminated intravascular coagulation (DIC) occurs frequently in a variety of patients, usually in subclinical forms that are handled well by the patient and so create no problems. However, it is important that chronic DIC (subclinical) be recognized, since these patients, if stressed hemostatically as in this case, can go on to develop serious problems that have to be managed clinically.

DIC is always secondary to some initiating event. With rare exceptions (some snake venoms), thrombin is generated. The point at which activation of either the intrinsic and/or extrinsic system is activated is variable. Thus, the most reproducible events to look for in the laboratory are the consequences of thrombin generation—that of platelet and fibrinogen consumption. Acute DIC usually presents no problem in diagnosis. In chronic DIC, where the stimulus may wax and wane in intensity, the parallel consumption of fibrinogen and platelets is often not as apparent. Fibrinogen is an acute phase protein, and the body's response to consumption is to increase synthesis so that, commonly, the fibrinogen in these patients is normal or even increased. Additionally, even though platelet production can rebound to some degree, platelets usually remain slightly below normal in chronic DIC.

The fibrinolytic system is always activated secondarily to thrombin generation, so evidence of this is also present. Most commonly, an elevated level of fibrin split products (fsp) will be seen. Again, in chronic DIC this may not be obvious; it is common to obtain equivocal or even normal results on this test. Soluble fibrin monomers (SFM) theoretically can be found. SFM are formed when thrombin splits fibrinogen (forming a fibrin monomer) in the presence of fsp. The fsp bind to the fibrin monomer, thus inhibiting the polymerization of these monomers. Hence, they are said to be "soluble." However, the test systems used in the literature for detection of the presence of SFM present difficulties in standardization and reproducibility so that a negative result may not be useful. A newer test, D-D dimers, seems to have the potential of improving detection of the consequences of fibrinolysis (review Section F, 5).

There is controversy about whether or not the diagnosis of primary fibrinolysis even exists. In theory, the fibrinolytic system is activated in the absence of a clotting stimulus. Hence, there is no thrombin generation, and therefore no soluble fibrin monomers or D-D dimers would be found. In addition, platelets are not consumed. However, since plasmin does degrade fibrinogen (as well as factors V and VIII and fibrin monomers and polymers), fibrinogen levels do decrease in primary fibrinolysis and fibrinogen split products are formed. Most of the test systems for fibrin split products equally detect fibrinogen split products. These tests will then also show an increased level in primary fibrinolysis.

Bibliography

Beck WS: Hematology, 3rd ed. Cambridge, MIT Press, 1981

Henry JB: Clinical Diagnosis and Management by Laboratory Methods, 17th ed. Philadelphia, WB Saunders, 1984

Murano G, Bick RL: Basic Concepts of Hemostasis and Thrombosis, 3rd ed. Philadelphia, Lea & Febiger, 1980

Sirridge MS, Shannon R: Laboratory Evaluation of Hemostasis and Thrombosis, 3rd ed. Philadelphia, WB Saunders, 1983

Thompson AR, Harker LA: Manual of Hemostasis and Thrombosis, 3rd ed. Philadelphia, FA Davis, 1983

Williams WJ: Hematology, 3rd ed. New York, McGraw-Hill, 1983

Case 3

A 19-YEAR-OLD BLACK WOMAN presents to her physician on January 25 with the complaint of nausea and vomiting. Her last normal menstrual period began on November 4. Physical examination of the patient shows her to be pregnant, with an expected date of confinement in August. She has had some intermittent dark spotting, but no major bleeding with associated cramping and passage of tissue. The remainder of the physical examination is unremarkable.

A routine urinalysis was performed with the following macroscopic examination results:

Appearance	= yellow, hazy	
Specific gravity	= 1.020	
pH	= 6.5	(5.0–8.0)
Protein	= neg	(neg)
Glucose	= neg	(neg)
Ketone	= neg	(neg)
Bilirubin	= neg	(neg)
Occult blood (nonhemolyzed)	= trace	(neg)
Nitrite	= neg	(neg)
Urobilinogen	= 0.1	(0.1–1.0)
WBC esterase	= neg	(neg)

Go to Section A.

Section A

A microscopic examination was done with the following results: squamous epithelium present, no crystals or bacteria noted. What would be the expected results for the following additional microscopic examination values?

WBC/High-Power Field (HPF)

(Select one.)

1. 20–50 (2+)

[   ]

2. Greater than 50, less than packed (3+)

[   ]

3. Less than 5 (occasional)

[   ]

RBC/HPF

(Select one.)

1. Negative

[   ]

2. 5–8 (1+)

[   ]

3. Greater than 30, less than packed (3+)

[   ]

Hyaline Casts/Low-Power Field (LPF)

(Select one.)

1. 5–10 (2+)

[   ]

2. Less than 1 (occasional)

[   ]

3. 1–5 (1+)

[   ]

Section B

A negative WBC esterase indicated the general absence of leukocytes.

Return to Section A.

Section C

A nonhemolyzed trace reading (occult blood) equates to the identification of approximately 5 to 8 intact red blood cells per high-power field in the microscopic examination.

Return to Section A.

Section D
An occasional hyaline cast can be a normal finding in an essentially negative urine specimen such as this. One to two leukocytes and a few squamous epithelial cells are considered normal. The trace amount of blood probably relates to the patient's spotting.

Go to Section E.

Section E
A complete blood cell count was performed with the following results:

White blood cells (WBC)	$= 8.1 \times 10^3/\mu l$	(4.0–10.0)
Red blood cells (RBC)	$= 4.29 \times 10^6/\mu l$	(4.20–5.40)
Hemoglobin (HGB)	= 10.2 g/dl	(11.5–15.5)
Hematocrit (HCT)	= 32%	(36–46)
Mean corpuscular volume (MCV)	= 75 femtoliter (fl)	(81–99)
Mean corpuscular hemoglobin (MCH)	= 23.9 picogram (pg)	(27.0–33.0)
Mean corpuscular hemoglobin concentration (MCHC)	= 31.7 g/dl	(31–35)

RBC Morphology
    Moderate microcytosis
    Hypochromia
    Slight polychromasia

Which of the following laboratory tests would be of value in helping to determine the cause of the microcytic, hypochromic red blood cell indices and anemia? (Select one.)

1. Vitamin B_{12} determination

   [   ]

2. Folic acid (folate) determination

   [   ]

3. Serum iron (serum Fe), total iron-binding capacity (TIBC), and percent transferrin saturation (% sat)

   [   ]

Section F
A significant number of women are iron deficient, and they may present with anemia and microcytic, hypochromic red blood cell indices. The patient in this case had the following iron status results:

Serum Fe	$= 91 \mu g/dl$	(40–160)
TIBC	$= 433 \mu g/dl$	(250–400)
% saturation	= 21%	(20–55)

Is the patient iron deficient?
    1. Yes
       [   ]
    2. No
       [   ]

Section G

The serum Fe in a normal adult ranges from 40 to 160 $\mu g/dl$, with 100 $\mu g/dl$ being an average normal value. This represents only about one-third of the binding capacity of transferrin so that the saturation % is about 30%. Both the serum Fe and the TIBC level are altered by disease states. Iron deficiency shows a major reduction in the serum Fe and a dramatic increase in the TIBC, often giving a saturation below 10%. In contrast, infection and inflammation reduce both the serum Fe and the TIBC. Pregnancy is associated with an increase in the TIBC.

Go to Section H.

Section H

Since this patient is not iron deficient, what might be another cause of the microcytic, hypochromic anemia? (Select one.)
    1. Anemia of chronic inflammation
       [   ]
    2. Vitamin B_{12} deficiency
       [   ]
    3. Thalassemia
       [   ]
    4. Folic acid deficiency
       [   ]

Section I

Most patients with the anemia of chronic inflammation have hemoglobin levels greater than 9.0 g/dl. The red cell morphology is normocytic or mildly microcytic with little or no anisocytosis. Shift cells (polychromasia) are not seen on the smear. The serum Fe and TIBC are reduced. Usually there is evidence of inflammation, including fever and leukocytosis.

Go back to Section H and select another alternative.

Section J

Patients with vitamin B_{12} deficiency usually have MCVs ranging between 100 to 140 fl with true macro-ovalocytes and prominent anisocytosis and poikilocytosis. The presence of some hypersegmented granulocytes is also highly suggestive; however, as a sole finding this is not pathognomonic for vitamin B_{12} deficiency. Pancytopenia is a usual finding.

Go back to Section H and select another alternative.

Section K

The term *thalassemia* refers to a heterogeneous group of hereditary disorders in which mutation leads to a quantitative reduction in globin synthesis. Typically, individuals present with microcytic or microcytic, hypochromic red blood cell indices. Heterozygotes either have no anemia or are mildly anemic, and the serum Fe studies are usually normal.

Go to Section M.

Section L

An individual with folic acid deficiency has the same hematopoietic profile as the person with vitamin B_{12} deficiency. A differential diagnosis may be made from clinical data; however, a biochemical diagnosis usually is done by specifically assaying the serum vitamin levels.

Go back to Section H and select another alternative.

Section M

Hemoglobin electrophoresis at alkaline pH was done. What would the expected hemoglobin pattern be in this case? (Select one.)

1. Hemoglobin A, S, A_2
   [   ]
2. Hemoglobin A, C
   [   ]
3. Hemoglobin A, A_2 increased
   [   ]
4. Hemoglobin A, A_2 decreased
   [   ]

Section N

Sickle cell trait appears almost exclusively in blacks and is benign when there are no complicating factors, such as coexistent iron deficiency or α-thalassemia. There is no associated anemia and the red blood cell indices are normal.

Go back to Section M and select another alternative.

Section O

Hemoglobin C trait appears almost exclusively in blacks and is benign when there are no complicating factors, such as coexistent iron deficiency or α-thalassemia. There is no associated anemia and the red blood cell indices are normal.

Go back to Section M and select another alternative.

Section P
The hemoglobin electrophoretic pattern in heterozygous β-thalassemia (β-thalassemia trait or β-thalassemia minor) typically consists of hemoglobin A, an elevated hemoglobin A_2 level, and about 50% of cases have a slight elevation of hemoglobin F. Heterozygous β-thalassemia is seen in approximately 1.5% of American blacks.

Go to Section R.

Section Q
In the adult, this electrophoretic pattern is consistent with iron deficiency. The iron studies in this case are normal, however, with the exception of the elevated TIBC, which is associated with pregnancy.

Go back to Section M and select another alternative.

Section R
What laboratory procedure should be done to confirm a diagnosis of β-thalassemia trait? (Select one.)

    1. Hemoglobin A_2 quantitation
      [   ]
    2. Reticulocyte index
      [   ]
    3. Indirect bilirubin
      [   ]

Section S
The main diagnostic feature of β-thalassemia trait is an elevated hemoglobin A_2 level in the 3.5%–7.0% range. The hemoglobin A_2 quantitation value in this patient was 5.0%.

Go to Section V.

Section T
The reticulocyte index (RI) is an approximate measure of effective red cell production, and an initial physiologic separation of anemias can be made by using this index as follows: hemolytic abnormalities >3, hypoproliferative and maturation abnormalities <2. The RI is calculated as follows:

$$\frac{\text{reticulocyte count \% } \times \text{ hematocrit correction}}{\substack{\text{2.0 (maturation time correction)} \\ \text{(if polychromasia is present)}}}$$

This patient had a 3.5% reticulocyte count and the

$$RI = \frac{3.5 \times \dfrac{32}{45}}{2.0} = 1.2$$

The thalassemias generally are classified as cytoplasmic maturation defect anemias; however, the RI alone cannot pinpoint a diagnosis.

Go back to Section R and select another alternative.

Section U
The indirect serum bilirubin level in this patient was 1.3 mg/dl. This is slightly elevated and reflects evidence of some increased red cell death during development. This can't be considered diagnostic of β-thalassemia trait, however, because indirect bilirubin levels may or may not be increased in this condition. Bilirubin excretion in the urine is not increased when there is an increased amount of indirect bilirubin in the circulation.

Go back to Section R and select another alternative.

Section V
In reviewing the initial hematological laboratory data in this case, which result is not typical of β-thalassemia trait? (Select one.)

1. MCV
   [   ]
2. MCH
   [   ]
3. HCT
   [   ]
4. RBC morphology
   [   ]
5. RBC
   [   ]

Section W
Studies show that adult black women with β-thalassemia trait have reduced MCVs in the 60 to 76 fl range.

Return to Section V.

Section X
Studies show that adult black women with β-thalassemia trait have reduced MCH values in the 18 to 24 pg range.

Return to Section V.

Section Y

Patients with heterozygous β-thalassemia typically have no anemia or are only mildly anemic. Studies show something other than thalassemia trait is ongoing when the hematocrit in women is <31%. The vast majority of individuals with β-thalassemia trait go through life without any complications that can be ascribed to the disease. The only complication of any importance is a worsening of anemia during pregnancy, and occasionally quite severe anemia may result.

Return to Section V.

Section Z

Microcytosis is the rule in β-thalassemia trait. There may or may not be hypochromia, target cells, and basophilic stippling. Slight to mild polychromasia may be present in some patients. Poikilocytosis is minimal and probably is overemphasized since the red cell distribution width (RDW) is usually normal.

Return to Section V.

Section AA

Mild erythrocytosis is common in β-thalassemia trait, with RBC counts in black females ranging from 5.03 to 5.86 × $10^6/\mu l$. The RBC count in this case is on the low side of normal. This is due to the hemodilution of pregnancy.

Go to the Enrichment Section.

Enrichment Section

The pathophysiology of β-thalassemia trait relates to one of two beta globin genes, which is replaced by a variant gene. This causes a decrease in overall beta chain production and a reduction in the amount of hemoglobin A formed $(\alpha_2\beta_2)$. The oversupply of alpha chains combines with delta chains to produce increased amounts of hemoglobin A_2 $(\alpha_2\delta_2)$ and in some cases increased amounts of hemoglobin F $(\alpha_2\gamma_2)$. Excess free alpha chains are very unstable and precipitate in the developing red cell in the bone marrow, causing early cell destruction. Typically this globin chain imbalance in the trait form is mild and there isn't excessive red blood cell destruction.

Beta-thalassemia trait is the thalassemic disorder most frequently found in North America and among Caucasians in general. It is of particularly high frequency among those of Mediterranean ancestry. Less well known is the fact that it occurs in almost all ethnic groups, as exemplified by this case.

Beta-thalassemia trait generally is an entirely innocuous condition and the patient with this finding should be reassured of its benignity.

Problems arise when a thalassemic gene is inherited from both parents, giving rise to β-thalassemia major, or when it is inherited together with a gene for an abnormal hemoglobin such as sickle/β-thalassemia. The most common problem in clinical practice is to distinguish heterozygous β-thalassemia from simple iron-deficiency anemia.

Bibliography
Fairbanks VF: Hemoglobinopathies and Thalassemias: Laboratory Methods and Case Studies. New York, Brian C Decker, 1980
Hillman RS, Finch CA: Red Cell Manual, 5th ed. Philadelphia, FA Davis, 1985
Weatherall DJ, Clegg JB: The Thalassemia Syndromes, 3rd ed. Oxford, Blackwell, 1981

Case 4

A 30-YEAR-OLD WHITE WOMAN was admitted with a 23-year history of Coombs'-positive hemolytic anemia. The first episode had occurred at the age of 7 years. Over the years she experienced periods of deep vein thrombosis and diffuse aching in the joints. Occasional bouts of pericarditis occurred and purpuric lesions on the arms and legs appeared at varying intervals.

On admission she presented with symptoms of weakness, fatigability, back pain, darkening of urine, low-grade fever, and headaches.

WBC (corrected for NRBC)	$= 11 \times 10^3/\mu l$	(4.0–10.0)
HCT	= 21%	(36–46)
MCV	= 134 fl	(81–99)
Nucleated red blood cell (NRBC)	= 57/100 WBC	
Platelet (PLT)	$= 82 \times 10^3/\mu l$	(150–450)

Differential
    41% neutrophils
    2% bands
    48% lymphocytes
    6% monocytes
    1% eosinophils

Reticulocyte count	= 37%	(Reticulocyte production index [RPI] 8.4%)

Morphology
    Howell-Jolly bodies
    Basophilic stippling
    Pappenheimer bodies
Urinalysis
    2+ protein
    4+ blood
    10–12 RBC/hpf

Coagulation
    PT 15.0 sec (11–14)
    Activated partial thromboplastin time (APTT) 70 sec (30–45)

The patient was put on prednisone (60 mg/day) until the hemolytic crisis subsided.

Go to Section A.

Section A
Which of the following additional tests would be helpful at this time? (Select three.)

    1. Antinuclear antibody (ANA)
        [   ]

    2. Serum complement level
        [
                                                              ]

    3. Bilirubin
        [
                                                              ]

    4. Lactic dehydrogenase (LD)
        [
                                                              ]

    5. Lupus erythematosus (LE) prep
        [   ]

Section B
ANA is a good screening test for this disease. It is sensitive although not specific.

Go to Section C.

Section C
The pattern of nuclear fluorescence is often associated with the type of antibody present. Choose the antibody that represents a peripheral pattern around the nucleus. (Select one.)

    1. Extractable nuclear antigen (ENA)
        [   ]

    2. Anti-DNA antibody
        [   ]

    3. Antibody to deoxyribonucleoprotein
        [   ]

    4. Nucleolar RNA
        [   ]

Section D

Which antibody is associated with the speckled nuclear pattern? (Select one.)

  1. Extractable nuclear antigen (ENA)
  [   ]
  2. Anti-DNA antibody
  [   ]
  3. Antibody to deoxyribonucleoprotein
  [   ]
  4. Nucleolar RNA
  [   ]

Section E

Which antibody is associated with the homogeneous nuclear pattern? (Select one.)

  1. Extractable nuclear antigen (ENA)
  [   ]
  2. Anti-DNA antibody
  [   ]
  3. Antibody to deoxyribonucleoprotein
  [   ]
  4. Nucleolar RNA
  [   ]

Section F

Which antibody is associated with the nucleolar pattern of fluorescence? (Select one.)

  1. Extractable nuclear antigen (ENA)
  [   ]
  2. Anti-DNA antibody
  [   ]
  3. Antibody to deoxyribonucleoprotein
  [   ]
  4. Nucleolar RNA
  [   ]

Section G

The LE prep may be helpful, although it is still not very specific. Select the necessary components for a positive LE prep. (Select four.)

  1. Intact lymphocytes
  [   ]

2. Intact neutrophils

[

]

3. Tart cells

[   ]

4. Damaged leukocytes

[

]

5. Platelets

[   ]

6. Complement

[

]

7. Antinucleoprotein IgG

[

]

Section H

Which tests would help confirm this diagnosis? (Select two.)

1. Anti–double-stranded (native) DNA

[

]

2. Anti–single-stranded (denatured) DNA

[   ]

3. Anti-Sm

[

]

4. Anti–nuclear ribonucleoprotein (RNP)

[   ]

5. Antibodies to cytoplasmic antigen Ro (SS-A)

[   ]

6. Anti-La (SS-B)

[   ]

Section I

Of the following, which disease best correlates with the laboratory test findings? (Select one.)

1. Mixed connective tissue disease (MCTD)
   [   ]

2. Sjögren's syndrome
   [   ]

3. Systemic lupus erythematosus (SLE)
   [   ]

4. Autoimmune hemolytic anemia (AIHA)
   [   ]

5. Fabry's disease
   [   ]

6. Rheumatoid arthritis
   [   ]

Section J

Select the age group that this disease normally affects. (Select one.)

1. Less than 10 years of age
   [   ]

2. 10–20 years of age
   [   ]

3. 20–30 years of age
   [   ]

4. Greater than 50 years of age
   [   ]

Section K

What is the female-to-male ratio for this disease? (Select one.)

1. 1 : 1
   [   ]

2. 1 : 2
   [   ]

3. 3 : 1
   [   ]

4. 9 : 1
   [   ]

Section L

What factors may precipitate exacerbation of this disease after a symptom-free period of time? (Review all choices.)

1. Drugs

[   ]

2. Physical and emotional stress

[   ]

3. Infections

[   ]

4. Surgery

[   ]

5. Pregnancy

[   ]

6. Exposure to the sun

[   ]

Section M

What is a possible explanation for the abnormal urine results associated directly with the disease? (Select one.)

1. Kidney infection

[   ]

2. Immune complexes in the glomeruli

[–   ]

3. Renal neoplasia

[   ]

4. Pyelonephritis

[   ]

Section N

Lupus nephritis presents in four stages of severity. What is the clinical feature of mesangial lupus nephritis, Stage I? (Select one.)

1. Proteinuria 4+

[   ]

2. Hematuria 3+

[   ]

3. No or minimal proteinuria and hematuria

[   ]

4. Casts (40 granular/lpf)

[   ]

Section O
What are the clinical features of focal proliferation nephritis, Stage II? (Select two.)

    1. Proteinuria 3+
    [   ]

    2. Hematuria 2+
    [   ]

    3. No clinical abnormalities
    [   ]

    4. Casts (10 waxy/lpf)
    [   ]

Section P
What are the clinical features of membranous lupus nephritis, Stage III? (Select two.)

    1. Nephrotic syndrome
    [   ]

    2. No clinical abnormalities
    [   ]

    3. Hypertension
    [   ]

Section Q
What are the clinical features of diffuse proliferative nephritis, the end stage kidney disease in lupus, Stage IV? (Review all choices.)

    1. Renal insufficiency
    [   ]

    2. Nephrotic syndrome
    [   ]

    3. Hypertension
    [   ]

Section R
Anemia in SLE is common. What are the causes of anemia? (Select all correct alternatives.)

    1. Anemia of chronic disease
    [   ]

    2. Autoimmune hemolytic anemia
    [   ]

    3. Marrow infarction and necrosis
    [   ]

4. Microangiopathic hemolytic anemia

[   ]

Section S

Anemia of chronic disease is the most common cause of anemia in SLE. It normally presents as a normochromic, normocytic anemia, although it may become hypochromic, microcytic. To distinguish anemia of chronic disease from iron-deficiency anemia (IDA), the following test results are found:

SLE
Decreased serum iron
Normal to decreased TIBC
Decreased % saturation
Normal to increased iron stores
Increased serum ferritin

IDA
Decreased serum iron
Increased TIBC
Decreased % saturation
Decreased iron stores
Decreased serum ferritin

Return to Section R.

Section T

This patient presented with an autoimmune hemolytic anemia (AIHA). The elevated WBC and increased MCV are related to this process. The elevated WBC is due to an increased hematopoiesis and stress. The increased MCV is due to the marked elevation of reticulocytes, although this is not a common occurrence in SLE. In AIHA, the antibodies responsible are usually of the "warm" type, reacting best at 37°C, and are IgG and/or IgM. In SLE, complement is always bound with the antibody. The AIHA is Coombs-positive and may precede the actual disease of SLE by years. SLE should be suspected if a young woman appears with an AIHA associated with complement and IgG. Idiopathic AIHA associated with other diseases usually does not bind complement.

Return to Section R.

Section U

The pancytopenia that SLE patients often present with suggests the possibility of antibodies to humoral marrow factors or immune complexes deposited in the vasculature resulting in marrow infarcts and necrosis. The exact degree of anemia produced by this mechanism is difficult to determine.

Return to Section R.

Section V

Microangiopathic hemolytic anemia may occur because of immune complexes laying down and altering the vasculature of the capillaries and small blood vessels, leading to a hemolytic state.

Go to Section W.

Section W
What additional test could be done to work up the abnormal coagulation tests? (Select one.)

    1. Fibrin split products

      [   ]

    2. Fibrin degradation products

      [   ]

    3. Factor assays

      [   ]

    4. Euglobulin lysis

      [   ]

    5. Fibrinogen

      [   ]

    6. Thrombin time

      [   ]

    7. Circulating anticoagulant

      [   ]

Section X
Factor assays may show a slight decrease in one or more of the factors but factor activity increases with additional dilutions of the patient's plasma. This occurs because there is less inhibitor neutralizing the phospholipid at higher dilutions. The only exception is factor II deficiency, which occurs in about 50% of patients with SLE with a lupus anticoagulant.

Return to Section W and select again.

Section Y
With the circulating anticoagulant correction studies, the lupus anticoagulant does not correct with the addition of normal plasma nor a progressive inhibition on incubation as is seen with most cases of other inhibitors. A factor deficiency will correct with the addition of normal plasma.

Go to Section Z.

Section Z
What are the factors a lupus anticoagulant could inhibit? (Select three.)

    1. Specific *in vivo* factor VIII

      [   ]

    2. Phospholipid

      [

3. Antithrombin III
[   ]

4. Cardiolipin

5. Activation of prothrombin by prothrombinase complex (Xa + Va + Ca^{++} + phospholipid)

Section AA

What tests could be used to identify a lupus-type anticoagulant? (Select one.)

1. Platelet neutralization procedure

2. Tissue thromboplastin inhibition test

3. Thrombin time
[   ]

Section BB

What clinical complications could be expected from the abnormal coagulation tests? (Select one.)

1. Thrombosis

2. Ecchymoses or purpura

3. Spontaneous bleeding
[   ]

4. No bleeding problems

Continued

Section CC
Why do SLE patients have an increased incidence of deep vein thrombosis? (Review all alternatives.)

1. Increase in clotting factors

2. Decreased antithrombin III

3. Decreased protein C

4. Decreased protein S

5. Inhibition of prostacyclin formation by endothelial cells

Section DD
What are the possible explanations for the purpura on this patient's extremities? (Select two.)

1. Thrombocytopenia

2. Acute vasculitis

3. Circulating anticoagulant

4. Factor deficiency

Section EE

Lupus is a disease of multiorgan involvement. What are some possible causes of the neurologic symptoms associated with SLE? (Review all alternatives.)

   1. Acute vasculitis

[

]

   2. Antineuronal cytoplasmic antibodies

[

]

   3. Deposition of immune complexes in the choroid plexus

[   ]

   4. Viral infection

[   ]

   5. Decreased hemostatic pressure

[   ]

Section FF

What may be an explanation for the intermittent joint pain described by the patient? (Review all alternatives.)

   1. Rheumatoid arthritis

[   ]

   2. Osteonecrosis

[

]

   3. Avascular necrosis

[

]

   4. Arthritis of SLE

[

]

Section GG

What will be the findings on a synovial fluid analysis in a patient with SLE? (Select one.)

   1. Increased PMN count of greater than $25 \times 10^3/\mu l$

[   ]

2. Poor mucin

[   ]

3. Glucose level increased

[

]

4. WBCs slightly increased, less than $3 \times 10^3/\mu l$, with the presence of lymphocytes and plasma cells

[

]

Section HH
The cardiac involvement can be associated with which of the following? (Select two.)

1. Libman-Sacks endocarditis

[

]

2. Myocarditis

[   ]

3. Myocardial infarct

[   ]

4. Congenital complete heart block

[   ]

Section II
What is the marker for high risk in neonatal lupus with a complete heart block? (Select one.)

1. Antinuclear antibodies

[-   ]

2. Anti-Sm

[   ]

3. Anti-Ro or anti-SS-A

[

]

Section JJ
What are the common symptoms that present in this disease but do not occur in this case study? (Select two.)

1. Butterfly rash

   [   ]

2. Dyspnea

   [   ]

3. Tachycardia

   [   ]

4. Blurred vision

   [   ]

5. Alopecia

   [   ]

Section KK

What symptoms are associated with an unfavorable prognosis? (Select two.)

1. Pericarditis

   [   ]

2. AIHA

   [   ]

3. Kidney disease

   [   ]

4. Central nervous system symptoms

   [   ]

5. Erythema

   [   ]

Section LL

What etiologic factors are implicated in SLE? (Review all alternatives.)

1. Genetic

   [   ]

2. Viral

   [   ]

3. Bacterial

[   ]

4. Immunologic factors

[   ]

Section MM

There is a strong association between some of the major histocompatibility complexes and SLE. These are:

HLA-DR2
HLA-DR3
HLA-A1
HLA-B8

Return to LL and select another alternative.

Section NN

There appears to be no direct cause documented in humans. However, viral infections can cause a disruption of the T suppressor cell population, which does at least implicate viruses in this disease.

Return to LL and select another alternative.

Section OO

There is a fundamental derangement of the immune system. Failure is of the immunoregulatory mechanisms that sustain self-tolerance.

Go to Section PP.

Section PP

What specific cells or factors are involved in the immunologic abnormalities? (Review all alternatives.)

1. T cells

[   ]

2. B cells

[   ]

3. PMNs

[

]

4. Monocytes

[

]

5. Drugs

[   ]

Section QQ

What functions or products of T cells are not normal? (Review all alternatives.)

    1. T-8 (T-suppressor) number

       [   ]

    2. T-8 function

       [   ]

    3. T-4 (T-helper) number

       [   ]

    4. T-4 function

       [   ]

    5. T cell response to interferon

       [   ]

Section RR

Whether exogenous or endogenous, the B cell is activated. This results in a heightened proliferative activity and the secretion of excessive immunogloblin against self and nonself.

Return to Section PP and review the next alternative.

Section SS

Select the drugs that can cause a drug-induced SLE. (Select three.)

    1. Aspirin

       [   ]

    2. Hydralazine

       [   ]

    3. Procainamide

       [   ]

    4. D-penicillamine

       [   ]

    5. Sulfonamides

       [   ]

Section TT

What is the mechanism of drug-induced SLE? (Select one.)

    1. Inhibition of ANA

       [   ]

   2. Inflammation of joints

[   ]

   3. Genetic

[   ]

Section UU

It is a genetically determined delay or inability to acetylate the amine or hydralazine moiety of these drugs. The malfunction is of the hepatic N-acetylate transferase system.

Go to Section VV.

Section VV

What is the treatment for drug-induced SLE? (Select one.)

   1. Remove the drug and the patient returns to normal.

[   ]

   2. Steroids

[   ]

   3. Immunosuppressive drugs

[   ]

   4. Salicylates

[   ]

Section WW

What therapy is most useful in treating SLE symptoms? (Review all alternatives.)

   1. Salicylates

[   ]

   2. Antimalarial drugs

[   ]

   3. Corticosteroids

[   ]

Section XX

What are the major causes of death? (Select two.)

   1. Infections

[   ]

2. Cardiovascular accident
   [   ]
3. Myocardial infarct
   [   ]
4. Renal disease
   [   ]
5. Hemorrhages
   [   ]

Section YY

The survival rate is directly associated with the degree of organ involvement, but what is the average survival for lupus patients? (Select one.)

1. 70% greater than 5 years
   [   ]
2. 50% greater than 5 years
   [   ]
3. 10% greater than 5 years
   [   ]
4. 5% greater than 5 years
   [   ]

Enrichment Section

The history of systemic lupus erythematosus has been recorded for over a hundred and forty years. It is a generalized inflammatory disease of the vascular and connective tissues. It has numerous multiorgan manifestations. The incidence is about 7/100,000 and has a young female predominance. The course of the disease can be intermittent, with extended periods of good health intermixed with episodes of active disease. Some patients may only demonstrate mild symptoms whereas others can run an acutely fatal course.

On examination the patient often presents with a characteristic facial butterfly rash, joint pain, and fever. The peripheral blood often shows a pancytopenia. The clinical manifestations can affect any organ system. Involvement of the renal system or nervous system seems to be associated with the poorest prognosis. Many clinical symptoms of SLE are due to tissue damage. The mechanism of this is directly related to the formation of autoantibody and immune complexes. The reticuloendothelial system, which normally removes immune complexes on formation, is not efficient and allows the build up and deposition of these complexes in the basement membranes of many organs. With this deposition the process of inflammation is initiated, leading to the pathogenic tissue damage found in SLE.

The disease has numerous etiologic aspects. There appears to be a genetic predisposition due to positive family histories. Viral involvement has been proven in mice and is strongly implicated as the agent that disrupts the normal immunity. The deranged immunity is associated with both T and B cells.

The best screening test for lupus is the ANA, which is positive in over 90% of patients with SLE. To confirm the diagnosis, the demonstration of native DNA and/or the Sm antigen gives the best definitive results.

Treatment is determined by the severity of the disease. Salicylates can treat the mild symptoms; antimalarial drugs help the skin rashes and arthritis symptoms; corticosteroids are reserved for the life-threatening manifestations. Hemolytic anemia and severe thrombocytopenia are usually the greatest concerns.

Life expectancy is directly related to the severity of the disease process. The range is from 0 to 20 years.

Bibliography

Barrett JT: Textbook of Immunology, 4th ed. St Louis, CV Mosby, 1983

Bennington JL: Dictionary and Encyclopedia of Laboratory Medicine and Technology. Philadelphia, WB Saunders, 1983

Harmon C: Antinuclear antibodies in autoimmune diseases. Med Clin North Am 69(3):547–559, 1985

Katz P: Clinical and laboratory evaluation of the immune system. Med Clin North Am 69(3):453–463, 1985

Lasser A: Serum antibodies in connective tissue diseases. Hum Pathol 12:1–4, 1981

Robbins SL, Cotran RS, Kimar V: Pathologic Basis of Disease, 3rd ed. Philadelphia, WB Saunders, 1984

Robinson DR: Systemic lupus erythematosus. Sci Am, 15 RHEVM Sect. IV, pp 1–14, 1984

Triplett DA: Hemostasis: A Case Oriented Approach. New York, Igaku-Shoin, 1984

Triplett DA: Laboratory Evaluation of Coagulation. Chicago, ASCP, 1982

Triplett DA: The laboratory heterogeneity of lupus anticoagulants. Arch Pathol Lab Med 109:946–950, 1984

Case 5

A 15-YEAR-OLD GIRL was brought to the emergency room with severe vomiting followed by signs of disturbed consciousness. Three days prior to the onset of vomiting she had recovered from an upper respiratory tract infection.

Section A

Select all preliminary laboratory data that would be helpful in pinpointing the cause of this patient's symptoms.

1. Electrolytes

[   ]

2. Aspartate aminotransferase (AST)

[   ]

3. Glucose

[   ]

4. Amylase

[   ]

5. Toxicology screen

[   ]

6. Cerebrospinal fluid (CSF)

[   ]

7. Blood/urine culture

[   ]

8. WBC

[   ]

Go to Section B.

Section B

Accumulated data reveal the preliminary problem to be which of the following? (Select one.)

1. Insulin shock
   [   ]
2. Encephalitis/meningitis
   [   ]
3. Salicylate intoxication
   [   ]
4. Hepatic dysfunction
   [   ]
5. Syndrome of inappropriate antidiuretic hormone (ADH) secretion
   [   ]

Section C

Clinical symptoms are suggestive of a hypoglycemic reaction, but blood glucose levels are only slightly decreased.

Return to Section B and select again.

Section D

Normal CSF findings and cultures help differentiate this condition from encephalitis/meningitis in which cell counts and protein would be abnormal.

Return to Section B and select again.

Section E

The toxicology screen revealed a salicylate level of 12 mg/dl. Symptoms from acute salicylate intoxication are usually not manifest until salicylate levels are 30 mg/dl.

Return to Section B and select again.

Section F

In order to better investigate the cause of the hepatic dysfunction, the following enzyme studies were done:

AST	= 1020 U/l (repeat)	(5–30)
Alanine aminotransferase (ALT)	= 885 U/l	(6–37)
Alkaline phosphatase (ALP)	= 110 U/l	(30–95)
LD	= 765 U/l	(80–280)
CK	= 620 U/l	(15–160)
GGT	= 28 U/l	(5–28)

These enzyme results are most suggestive of which disorder? (Select one.)

1. Acute viral hepatitis
   [   ]
2. Reye's syndrome
   [   ]
3. Biliary obstruction
   [   ]
4. Acute toxic hepatitis
   [   ]

Section G

The syndrome of inappropriate ADH secretion leads to excess ADH, which results in retention of water causing a volume expansion and dilutional hyponatremia. Sodium and chloride levels would characteristically be decreased instead of elevated.

Return to Section B and select again.

Section H

In acute hepatitis, the GGT level would typically be increased due to its sensitivity as an indicator of hepatocellular damage. CK would be normal due to its absence in liver tissue.

Return to Section F and select again.

Section I

These enzyme results are typical findings in Reye's syndrome. Extreme elevations can be found with AST, ALT, LD, and CK. ALP is usually only slightly elevated or normal and GGT is usually normal.

Go to Section L.

Section J

ALP levels are typically more predominantly elevated in biliary obstruction than are AST or ALT. Extreme increases in AST/ALT are not seen. GGT would be elevated due to its sensitivity as an indicator of hepatobiliary dysfunction. CK would be normal due to its absence in the liver or bile ducts.

Return to Section F and select again.

Section K

The enzyme picture in acute toxic hepatitis is similar to that in acute viral hepatitis. GGT would typically be increased due to its sensitivity as an indicator of hepatocellular damage. CK would be normal due to its absence in liver tissue.

Return to Section F and select again.

Section L

If AST isoenzyme studies were performed, which fraction would be most predominant? (Select one.)

      1. Cytoplasmic AST
        [   ]

      2. Mitochondrial AST
        [   ]

Section M

The normal isoenzyme ratio of cytoplasmic to mitochondrial AST ranges from 5:1 to 20:1. This ratio has been found to be reversed in Reye's syndrome due to the consequent mitochondrial injury that is characteristic of Reye's syndrome. Determination of the cytoplasmic-to-mitochondrial ratio may prove to have diagnostic value in differentiating Reye's syndrome from acute viral hepatitis, chronic aggressive hepatitis, acute fulminant hepatitis, and cirrhosis.

Go to Section N.

Section N

Reye's syndrome frequently presents with an acid/base imbalance. Blood gas studies were performed, with the following results:

pH = 7.52   (7.35–7.45)
pCO_2 = 27 mm Hg (35–45)
HCO_3 = 20 mmol/l (22–28)
pO_2 = 88 mm Hg (75–100)

    These results are characteristic of which type of acid/base disturbance? (Select one.)

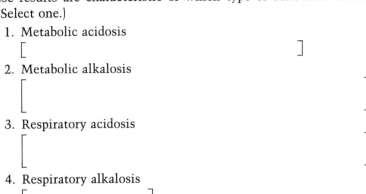

      1. Metabolic acidosis

      2. Metabolic alkalosis

      3. Respiratory acidosis

      4. Respiratory alkalosis

Section O

These results represent a respiratory alkalosis partially compensated by a metabolic acidosis. The acid/base abnormalities in Reye's syndrome are very complex and characteristically present as respiratory alkalosis and metabolic acidosis of varying degrees. Contributing factors include recurrent vomiting, dehydration, hyperventilation, salicylate intoxication, and organic acidemia.

Go to Section P.

Section P

Of the following tests, select the most useful abnormal finding in the diagnosis of Reye's syndrome. (Select one.)

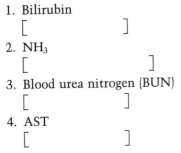

1. Bilirubin
   [   ]
2. NH_3
   [   ]
3. Blood urea nitrogen (BUN)
   [   ]
4. AST
   [   ]

Section Q

The blood ammonia concentration is typically elevated severalfold and is the major clue to the metabolic abnormalities of Reye's syndrome. Levels from 250 to 1000 $\mu g/dl$ (0–50) can be observed. Hyperammonemia most probably reflects hepatic dysfunction—specifically a disturbance in the urea cycle. The hyperammonemia is transient and returns to normal with or without treatment 24 to 72 hours after admission.

Go to Section R.

Section R

Select all other results that are likely to be abnormal in Reye's syndrome.

1. BUN
   [   ]
2. Prothrombin time
   [   ]
3. CK isoenzymes
   [   ]
4. Bilirubin
   [   ]
5. Lipids/lipoproteins
   [   ]

Section S

BUN values ranging from normal to markedly increased (14–291 mg/dl) have been reported. Even though there is a block in the urea cycle that interferes with the synthesis of urea, it appears that this block is incomplete or capable of being partially overridden when increased substrate is present from increased protein catabolism. Therefore, BUN values are frequently elevated.

Return to Section R and select again.

Section T

Hypoprothrombinemia is seen in more than 50% of patients and probably accounts for the gastrointestinal bleeding that may occur. Deficient clotting factors are those synthesized in the liver.

Return to Section R and select again.

Section U

All four isoenzymes of CK have been reported: CK-MM, CK-MB, CK-BB, and mitochondrial CK. However, the presence of CK-BB is a rare finding. The bulk of the cathodic band may be due to mitochondrial CK, which would correlate with the widespread mitochondrial injury that occurs in Reye's syndrome.

Return to Section R and select again.

Section V

Bilirubin levels are typically normal or only slightly elevated despite the hepatic dysfunction characteristic of the disorder. Elevations above 2 mg/dl occur in only 20% of patients.

Return to Section R and select again.

Section W

Typical lipid/lipoprotein findings reveal elevations of free fatty acids, normal triglyceride levels, decreased total cholesterol concentration, and hypolipoproteinemia, particularly hypo-beta and hypo-alpha or an-alpha-lipoproteinemia. These findings are attributed, in part, to excessive lipolysis and impaired lipoprotein synthesis. The triglyceride synthetic pathway appears to be unaffected.

Go to the Enrichment Section.

Enrichment Section

Reye's syndrome is a rapidly progressive illness usually seen in children between the ages of 1 and 16 years. It is described as a syndrome of encephalopathy and fatty degeneration of the viscera, especially the liver.

In most patients the onset of the disorder follows a viral infection. Apparent recovery from the viral illness is followed by a sudden onset of vomiting and the appearance of neurological symptoms progressing from irritability and restlessness to delirium, stupor, and coma within the next 24 to 48 hours.

A major factor in the pathophysiology of the disease is mitochondrial injury in liver, muscle, and brain. The specific mitochondrial injury affects the initial, enzymatic steps of urea synthesis, resulting in extreme elevations of blood ammonia. A further insult of the mitochondrial injury is uncoupling of oxidative phosphorylation with resultant impairment of processes dependent on ATP. Processes affected include synthesis of apoproteins, vitamin K-dependent coagulation factors, and glycogen, and the maintenance of cell membrane integrity. These factors account, in part, for the abnormalities seen in levels of lipoproteins, prothrombin time, glucose, and the transaminases.

Fatty degeneration of the viscera, especially the liver, is a second major finding of Reye's syndrome in addition to mitochondrial injury. Lipid accumulates in the liver as a result of excessive lipolysis and mobilization of fatty acids, which are converted to triglycerides.

Blood ammonia levels begin to elevate in the initial stages of the disorder and usually decline rapidly after admission regardless of the outcome. Blood ammonia is usually normal at the time of death and is not the immediate cause of death.

Death often occurs as a result of excessive intracranial pressure due to disturbances in water and electrolyte balance attributed to an acute, irreversible lesion of the brain.

Bibliography
Brown RE, Forman DT: The biochemistry of Reye's syndrome. CRC Crit Rev Clin Lab Sci 17(1):247–297, 1982
Devivo DC, Keating JP: Reye's syndrome. Adv Pediatr 22:175, 1976
Reye RDK, Morgan G, Baral J: Encephalopathy and fatty degeneration of the viscera. Lancet 2:749–752, 1963

Case 6

A 54-YEAR-OLD WHITE MAN entered the hospital with the complaint of a degenerating racquetball game due to fatigue. On examination, the patient appeared pale, and he had had a recent weight loss of 15 pounds. Urinalysis results were within normal limits. CBC results were as follows:

WBC   = 3.4 × 10³/μl   (4.0–10.0
RBC   = 2.8 × 10⁶/μl   (4.20–5.40)
HGB   = 10.5 g/dl   (13.5–16.0)
HCT   = 32%   (36–46)
MCV   = 112 fl   (81–99)
MCH   = 36.8 pg   (27.0–33.0)
MCHC = 32.8 g/dl   (31–35)
PLT   = 178 × 10³/μl   (150–450)
Differential
    52% neutrophils
     1% bands
    35% lymphocytes
     1% eosinophils
    10% monocytes
     1% blasts
WBC morphology
    Degranulated neutrophils
    Pseudo Pelger-Huët anomaly
    Enlarged and bizarre platelet forms
RBC morphology
    Few macro-ovalocytes
Bone marrow differential
    10% blasts
     5% promyelocytes
     3% myelocytes
    20% metamyelocytes
     8% bands

15% neutrophils
2% lymphocytes
4% pronormoblasts
4% basophilic normoblasts
20% polychromatic normoblasts
9% orthochromatic normoblasts
Myeloid : erythroid (M : E) ratio = 1.6 : 1
Iron stain—8% ringed sideroblasts (type III)
Reticulin stain—1+
Comments on bone marrow
    Hypercellular
    Dyserythropoiesis
    Dysmyelopoiesis
    Dysmegakaryopoiesis

Go to Section A.

Section A
What condition would best correlate with the above findings? Identify by the French-American-British (FAB) classification. (Review all options.)

1. Refractory anemia (RA)
   [   ]

2. Refractory anemia with ringed sideroblasts (RARS, IRSA, IASA)
   [   ]

3. Refractory anemia with excess blasts (RAEB)
   [   ]

4. Chronic myelomonocytic leukemia (CMML)
   [   ]

5. Refractory anemia with excess blasts in transformation (RAEBIT)
   [   ]

Section B
RA is usually found in patients over 50 years of age. The peripheral blood shows an anemia with no other cytopenias. The anemia is dimorphic, meaning it can be macrocytic to microcytic and normochromic to hypochromic. These patients have a reticulocytopenia. The WBCs and platelets are usually normal. Bone marrow findings show erythroid hyperplasia with dyserythropoiesis, normocellularity or hypercellularity, and sideroblasts <15%. The granulopoiesis and megakaryopoiesis are basically normal. Blasts do not exceed 5%.

Go back to Section A and review the next option.

Section C

Refractory anemia with ringed sideroblasts has the same findings as RA (see Section B) except for the changes in the bone marrow. RARS has greater than 15% of type III ringed sideroblasts. A type III sideroblast has five or more siderotic granules covering one-third or more of the circumference of the nucleus. The granulopoiesis and megakaryopoiesis are still basically normal. Blasts do not exceed 5%.

Go back to Section A and review the next option.

Section D

Chronic myelomonocytic leukemia has the abnormalities found in RAEB (see Section F) plus greater than $1000/\mu l$ monocytes in the peripheral blood. Blasts do not exceed 5% in the peripheral blood or 20% in the bone marrow. Bone marrow resembles RAEB except for a pronounced increase in promonocytes and monocytes.

Go back to Section A and review the next option.

Section E

RAEBIT shows dysplasia in all three cell lines but the blast count in the bone marrow is now between 20% and 30% and Auer rods may be present. The peripheral blood shows cytopenias and greater than 5% blasts. Blasts may be type I or II (see Section F).

Go to Section G.

Section F

RAEB shows all the red cell changes found in RA or RARS (see Sections B and C, respectively) plus cytopenias affecting two or more cell lines. Peripheral blood shows less than 5% blasts of type I or II and no Auer rods. Dysmyelopoiesis is evident in the granulocytes. The bone marrow shows evidence of dyserythropoiesis, dysmyelopoiesis, and dysmegakaryopoiesis. The marrow is usually hypercellular. Type I and type II blasts range from 5% to 20%. The type I blast is a primitive cell with a central nucleus; nucleoli are present, and the cell has a fine chromatin pattern. The nuclear : cytoplasmic (N : C) ratio is high and no granules are present in the cytoplasm. The type II blast has a central nucleus, nucleoli, and a fine chromatin pattern. The N : C ratio is high and there may be abnormal primary granules in the cytoplasm that appear large or fused. These are not identical to normal promyelocytes. No Auer rods are present in the blasts. Serial maturation of the granulocytic precursors is present.

Go back to Section A and review the next option.

Section G

Select the changes that are associated with dyserythropoiesis. (Review all options.)

1. RBC multinuclearity

   [   ]

2. RBC nuclear fragmentation

   [   ]

3. Megaloblastoid changes

   [   ]

4. Megaloblastic changes

   [   ]

5. Vacuolated cytoplasm

   [   ]

6. Vacuolated nucleus

   [   ]

7. Nuclear bridging

   [   ]

8. Lobulated nuclei

   [   ]

9. Abnormal mitotic figures

   [   ]

10. Increased marrow iron with ringed sideroblasts

    [   ]

11. Resynthesis of fetal hemoglobin

    [   ]

Section H

Select the changes that are associated with dysmyelopoiesis. (Review all options.)

    1. Hypogranulation of neutrophils

[

]

    2. Pseudo Pelger-Huët anomaly

[

]

    3. Pseudo Chediak-Higashi syndrome

[

]

    4. Ring or rodent nuclei

[   ]

Section I

Select the changes that are associated with dysmegakaryopoiesis. (Review all options.)

    1. Micromegakaryocytes

[

]

    2. Circulating megakaryoblasts

[

]

    3. Nuclei with separated lobes

[

]

    4. Mononuclear forms

[

]

    5. Defective platelet production

[

]

    6. Enlarged platelets

[

]

7. Abnormal platelet granulation

[   ]

8. Vacuolated cytoplasm

[   ]

Section J
Select other names used for myelodysplastic syndromes. (Review all options.)

1. Smoldering acute leukemia

[   ]

2. Subacute myeloid leukemia

[   ]

3. Preleukemic syndrome

[   ]

4. Hematopoietic dysplasia

[   ]

Section K
What leukemias are *not* associated with a preleukemic phase? (Select four.)

1. M-1

[   ]

2. M-2 t(8 : 21)

[   ]

3. M-3 t(15 : 17)

[   ]

4. M-4

[   ]

5. M-5

[   ]

6. M-6

[   ]

7. ALL

[   ]

8. Philadelphia chromosome–positive acute leukemias

[   ]

Section L

What is the treatment of choice for RAEB? (Select one.)

1. Chemotherapy
   [   ]

2. Supportive therapy
   [   ]

3. Irradiation
   [   ]

4. Bone marrow transplant
   [   ]

Section M

It has not been proven to be beneficial to the patient to treat the disease aggressively with irradiation or chemotherapy. The treatment of choice is to respond to the symptoms that are usually related to the cytopenias. RBCs are transfused for severe anemia, platelets are transfused for thrombocytopenia, and antibiotic therapy is used to respond to infections due to neutropenia.

Go to Section N.

Section N

Sixteen months later, the patient was readmitted with fever, bleeding gums, and recurring nosebleeds. CBC results were as follows:

WBC = 142.3 × $10^3/\mu l$ (4.0–10.0)
HGB = 7.7 g/dl   (13.5–16.0)
MCV = 106 fl   (81–99)
PLT = 93 × $10^3/\mu l$ (150–400)
Differential
    12% neutrophils
    2% bands
    86% blasts
Comments on bone marrow
    Hypercellular
    90%–95% blasts (wipeout)

What further testing should be done at this point? (Review all alternatives.)

1. Cytochemistry
   [   ]

2. Cytogenetics
   [   ]

3. Monoclonal antibodies
   [   ]

Section O
Results of special stains:

Combined chloroacetate esterase and alpha napthol acetate esterase—positive for both
PAS—negative
Sudan black—moderate positivity
Peroxidase—moderate positivity

According to the results obtained on the special stains, which leukemia is indicated? (Select one.)

1. M-1 (acute myelogeneous leukemia without maturation)
   [   ]
2. M-2 (acute myelogenous leukemia with maturation)
   [   ]
3. M-3 (acute progranulocytic leukemia)
   [   ]
4. M-4 (acute myelomonocytic leukemia)
   [   ]
5. M-5a (acute monocytic leukemia, undifferentiated)
   [   ]
6. M-5b (acute monocytic leukemia, differentiated)
   [   ]
7. M-6 (erythroleukemia)
   [   ]

Section P
Cytogenetic studies were negative in this patient. This particular leukemia does not have cytogenetic findings that are clinically significant, although some leukemias have cytogenetic findings that have diagnostic and prognostic significance. Examples are the Philadelphia chromosome that is associated with 90% of the CMLs, the t(8:21) that is associated with M-2, and the t(15:17) that is associated with M-3.

Go back to Section N and review the next option.

Section Q
The use of the monoclonal antibodies for the acute nonlymphocytic leukemias (ANLL) have not been as significant clinically as those developed for the lymphoid cell line. The monoclonals for lymphocytic malignancies have proven prognostic significance. The monoclonals may help differentiate lymphoid from nonlymphoid malignancies.

Go to Section R.

Section R

Select clinical complications that could be manifest in this patient. (Review all options.)

1. Hyperviscosity

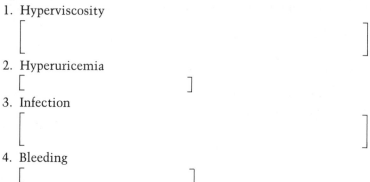

2. Hyperuricemia

3. Infection

4. Bleeding

Section S

Hyperuricemia is due to excessive cellular turnover. The normal secretion of uric acid in the urine is 300 to 500 mg/day. The excretion of this can increase up to 50 times normal in leukemia. Antileukemic therapy causes a dramatic increase in nucleic acid catabolism due to cell death. At an alkaline pH, the urates are soluble and at an acid pH they are insoluble. Therefore, the patient should be hydrated to keep the urine at an alkaline pH. In addition, the drug allopurinol inhibits xanthine oxidase, the enzyme that converts xanthine and hypoxanthine to uric acid during purine catabolism. Uric acid causes kidney damage, while xanthine is cleared by other mechanisms leaving the kidney undamaged.

Go back to Section R and review the next option.

Section T

Select the mechanisms that are involved in leukemia that can cause the patient to bleed. (Review all options.)

1. Thrombocytopenia

2. DIC

3. Leukemic infiltration

[

]

4. Leukostasis

[ ]

Section U
Depending on the cell size, high white blood cell counts of greater than 100 to 200 $\times$ $10^3/\mu l$ are capable of plugging the small vessels in the brain and causing hemorrhage. Another mechanism is that blasts migrate out of the vascular system and form nodules in the perivasculature adjacent to the blood vessel. The nodules grow and eventually rupture the vessel, causing hemorrhage.

Go to section V.

Section V
Select the mechanism that creates the cytopenias in acute leukemias. (Select one.)

1. LIA (leukemia-associated inhibition activity)

[

]

2. NRF (neutrophil-releasing factors)

[

]

3. BPA (burst-promoting activity)

[

]

4. PGE_1

[

]

Section W
Select factors that give leukemic cells the neoplastic growth advantage. (Select three.)

1. Autonomous production (insensitive to normal inhibitors)

[ ]

2. Extrasensitivity to CSA (colony-stimulating activity)

[ ]

3. All cells in a constant cell cycle

[

]

4. Rapid proliferation

[   ]

5. The leukemic cells lack the ability to mature but retain the ability to divide.

[

]

Section X

What is the incidence of leukemia in the United States? (Select one.)

1. 3.5 per 100,000

[   ]

2. 8.5 per 100,000

[   ]

3. 1.0 per 100,000

[   ]

Section Y

Select the etiologic factors involved in leukemia. (Review all options.)

1. Ionizing radiation

[

]

2. Toxic chemicals

[

]

3. Acquired hematologic diseases

[

]

4. Genetic

[

]

5. Viral

[

]

Section Z

Select the treatments used for acute myelomonocytic leukemia or any of the ANLL. (Review all options.)

1. Chemotherapy

[   ]

2. Bone marrow transplants

[   ]

3. Immunotherapy

[   ]

4. Maturation agents

[   ]

Enrichment Section

Acute leukemia is a malignant hematopoietic disease in which normal hematopoietic marrow is replaced by abnormal immature precursors. Leukemic cell production takes place in any organ capable of cell production. Hematopoiesis, whether normal or abnormal (leukemic), is clonal. The production of the clone originates in a stem cell that is able to maintain the clone by its capacity for self-renewal. A leukemogenic agent or stimulant alters DNA and forces certain genetic alterations.

Leukemic cells have varying abnormal presentations of proliferation and differentiation, which give us the subclasses in acute nonlymphocytic leukemia. M-1, M-2, and M-3 show different levels of maturation. M-4, M-5, and M-6 show proliferative alterations involving other cell lines.

The predominance of leukemic cells is due to their inhibition of normal hematopoiesis and the arrest in maturation in the mitotic compartment, allowing for a steady expansion of the leukemic cell line.

Diagnosis between ANLL and ALL is important because of the different chemotherapy regimens used in treatment. The ANLLs basically all use the same antitumor drugs, the most common being daunorubicin, cytosine arabinoside, and 6-thioguanine. Remission induction is the effort to decrease the tumor burden to the point that normal hematopoiesis can function again. Remission is defined as going from a leukemic cell population of $10^{12}/L$ to $10^9/L$. At $10^9/L$, normal hematopoiesis is able to function again. Duration of remissions only ranges from 10 to 15 months for ANLLs.

Bibliography

Golde D, Cline MJ: Regulation of granulopoiesis. N Engl J Med 291:1388–1395, 1974

Gunz F, Henderson E: Leukemia, 4th ed. New York, Grune & Stratton, 1983

Hayhoe FG, Quaglino D: Haematological Cytochemistry. London, Churchill Livingstone, 1980

Koepke JA: Laboratory Hematology. New York, Churchill Livingstone, 1984

Kushner J: Hematopoietic stem cell proliferation. Lab Med 12:279–282, 1981

Pierre R: Acute Nonlymphocytic Leukemias. ASCP Teleconferences, April, 1983

Pierre R: Myelodysplastic Syndromes. ASCP Teleconferences, May, 1983

Williams W: Hematology, 3rd ed. New York, McGraw-Hill, 1983

Wintrobe M: Clinical Hematology, 8th ed. Philadelphia, Lea & Febiger, 1981

Case 7

A 36-YEAR-OLD CAMBODIAN WOMAN who had been living in the United States for approximately two years was seen in the refugee clinic with complaints of chronic headache, insomnia, and right lower quadrant pain. Her general physical examination was normal with the exception of moderate right lower quadrant tenderness to deep palpation, without rebound. Screening laboratory tests, including a blood cell count with platelets and smear evaluation, an erythrocyte sedimentation rate (ESR), and routine urinalysis, were ordered with the following results:

WBC   = 4.0 × 10³/μl   (4.0–10.0)
RBC   = 4.63 × 10⁶/μl   (4.2–5.40)
HGB   = 11.7 g/dl   (11.5–15.5)
HCT   = 36%   (36–46)
MCV   = 78 fl   (81–99)
MCH   = 25.3 pg   (27.0–33.0)
MCHC = 32.6 g/dl   (31–35)
PLT   = 218 × 10³/μl   (150–450)
ESR   = 17 mm/hr   (0–20)
Smear evaluation
    RBC morphology
        Microcytosis
        Slight hypochromia
        Occasional target cells
    WBC morphology
        Normal
    PLT morphology
        Normal
Routine urinalysis, macroscopic examination
    Appearance   = normal
    Specific gravity = 1.022
    pH   = 5.0   (5.0–8.0)

Protein	= neg	(neg)
Glucose	= neg	(neg)
Ketones	= neg	(neg)
Bilirubin	= neg	(neg)
Occult blood	= neg	(neg)
Nitrite	= neg	(neg)
Urobilinogen	= 0.1	(0.1–1.0)
WBC esterase	= neg	(neg)

Routine urinalysis, microscopic examination

Occasional squamous epithelial cells, calcium oxalate crystals, and mucous threads present

Go to Section A

Section A

The borderline low hematocrit and microcytic red blood cell indices prompted the ordering of iron studies. A zinc protoporphyrin : heme ratio (ZnPP/heme) was done with the following result:

ZnPP/heme = 62 μmol/mol heme (<80)

Does this suggest iron-deficiency anemia? (Select one.)

    1. Yes

      [   ]

    2. No

      [   ]

Section B

The level of zinc erythrocyte protoporphyrin reflects the amount of protoporphyrin in excess of that used for hemoglobin synthesis. Levels greater than 80 μmol/mol heme are seen with iron-deficient erythropoiesis whether due to absolute iron deficiency or inflammation. Increased protoporphyrin also occurs with lead poisoning and certain rare disorders of porphyrin metabolism such as red cell protoporphyria. Changes in the red cell protoporphyrin take 2 to 3 weeks of sustained iron deficiency. Therefore, it is a more stable measure of chronic iron deficiency, in contrast to the serum iron, which can be depressed within hours due to a transient infection. In addition, erythrocyte protoporphyrin measures the level of iron supply relative to the need of the individual red cell.

Go to Section C.

Section C

An evaluation of the case at this point suggests a further need to investigate the following: (Review all choices.)

    1. Cause of right lower quadrant pain

      [   ]

2. Presence of infection

   [   ]

3. Cause of chronic headaches and insomnia

   [   ]

4. Presence of microcytic red blood cell indices

   [   ]

Section D

Further examination for the cause of the right lower quadrant pain revealed a mildly enlarged fibroid uterus. There were no adnexal masses.

Go back to Section C and review the next choice.

Section E

A review of the physical findings and results of the laboratory screening tests does not indicate the presence of infection. More specifically, expected laboratory results in infection might be an abnormal WBC count, elevated ESR, possibly abnormal WBC morphology, positive urine nitrite and WBC esterase results, with bacteria and WBCs present in the urine sediment, and an elevated ZnPP/heme ratio.

Go back to Section C and review the next choice.

Section F

The patient, at presentation, indicated that she had been depressed for some months. The chronic headaches and insomnia were thought to be tension-related as well as being associated with her depressed state. Medication was prescribed and she was asked to return to the clinic for follow-up in three weeks.

Go back to Section C and review the next choice.

Section G

Iron deficiency was ruled out as a cause of microcytosis. Thalassemia and thalassemia-like disorders also can cause microcytosis. An initial screening procedure for thalassemia is hemoglobin electrophoresis.

Go to Section H.

Section H

Cellulose acetate hemoglobin electrophoresis (pH 8.6) was performed on a sickle cell trait control (AS) and on the patient's blood sample. The results are shown in Figure 1. Hemoglobin S is a beta-chain variant and its concentration in AS is approximately 40% of the total hemoglobin. Hemoglobin A_2 values range between 2.3% to 4.3%, with a mean of 3.6% in the presence of hemoglobin S.

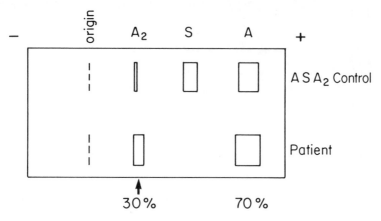

Figure 1

What hemoglobin(s) migrate(s) to the point indicated by the arrow on alkaline electrophoresis? (Review all choices.)

1. HGB D
   [   ]
2. HGB G
   [   ]
3. HGB C
   [   ]
4. HGB O$_{Arab}$
   [   ]
5. HGB A$_2$
   [   ]
6. HGB E
   [   ]

Section I

Hemoglobins D and G have mobilities that are indistinguishable from hemoglobin S at alkaline pH. The most common of these two variants are D$_{Los Angeles}$, usually found in whites, and G$_{Philadelphia}$, which is almost always limited to blacks. Hemoglobin D$_{Los Angeles}$ is a beta-chain variant and it coexists with hemoglobin A in a ratio of approximately 1 : 1. Hemoglobin G$_{Philadelphia}$ is an alpha-chain variant and it commonly is found in a ratio (to hemoglobin A) of 1 : 3, although this is variable.

Go back to Section H and review the next choice.

Section J
Hemoglobins C, O_{Arab}, A_2, and E all migrate to the area indicated by the arrow in Figure 1. What procedure can be done to begin to differentiate these hemoglobins? (Select one.)

1. Solubility test
   [   ]

2. Cellulose acetate electrophoresis at neutral pH
   [   ]

3. Acid elution slide test
   [   ]

4. Citrate agar electrophoresis
   [   ]

Section K
A positive solubility test confirms the presence of a sickling hemoglobin that may or may not be hemoglobin S. Most hemoglobins, including D, O_{Arab}, A_2, and E, give negative results.

Go back to Section J and select another alternative.

Section L
Cellulose acetate electrophoresis at neutral pH is done to separate hemoglobin H and hemoglobin Bart's from other fast-migrating hemoglobins. This procedure doesn't differentiate among hemoglobins C, O_{Arab}, A_2, and E.

Go back to Section J and select another alternative.

Section M
The acid elution slide test is done to determine the presence of hemoglobin F in red blood cells. It is not useful in making the differentiation among hemoglobins C, O_{Arab}, A_2, and E.

Go back to Section J and select another alternative.

Section N
Citrate agar electrophoresis (pH 6.2) clearly separates hemoglobins F, A, S, and C. Almost all other hemoglobins migrate close to or with hemoglobin A. The patient's sample was electrophoresed on agar and had one band in the hemoglobin A position as shown in Figure 2. This rules out hemoglobin C. Hemoglobin O_{Arab} migrates between A and S on citrate agar. Hemoglobins E and A_2 migrate with hemoglobin A.

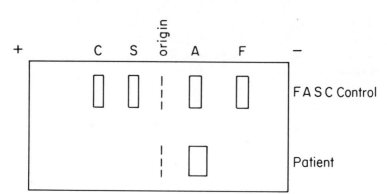

Figure 2

What differentiation can be made between hemoglobin E and A_2 at this point? (Select one.)

      1. The hemoglobin at the point of the arrow in Figure 1 is hemoglobin A_2 only.

      [   ]

      2. The hemoglobin at the point of the arrow in Figure 1 is hemoglobin E + A_2.

      [   ]

Section O

Hemoglobin A_2 can be accurately quantified and a reference range, using microchromatographic procedures, is approximately 1.9% to 3.2%. The concentration of hemoglobin A_2 alone is almost never higher than 10%.

Go back to Section N and select another alternative.

Section P

Hemoglobin E and A_2 migrate together at alkaline pH, and the hemoglobin E + A_2 concentration in hemoglobin E trait (AE) ranges from 27% to 35%.

Go to Section Q.

Section Q

The diagnosis of hemoglobin E trait was made. Why does the patient have microcytic indices? (Select one.)

      1. Hemoglobin E trait and alpha-thalassemia trait are coincident in this patient.

      [   ]

      2. A sampling error occurred.

      [   ]

3. Hemoglobin E trait is a thalassemia-like disorder.

[   ]

Section R
Alpha-thalassemia is prevalent in Southeast Asians, and when it coexists with hemoglobin E, the quantitation of hemoglobin E + A_2 is usually less than 27%.

Go back to Section Q and select another alternative.

Section S
The blood sample was properly drawn, the Coulter Counter was in calibration, and controls were valid.

Go back to Section Q and select another alternative.

Section T
Hemoglobin E (HGB E, $\alpha_2\beta_2$ ^{26}Glu → Lys) is a beta-chain variant; yet in hemoglobin E trait, it constitutes only about 30% of the total hemoglobin. Ribosomal synthesis of B^E-globin is decreased as compared with B^A-globin production, and thus a mild thalassemic blood picture with microcytosis results.

Go to Section U.

Section U
Is hemoglobin E trait a contributor to this patient's presenting complaints? (Select one.)

1. Yes

[   ]

2. No

[   ]

Section V
Individuals with hemoglobin E trait typically have no clinical symptoms.

Go to Section W.

Section W
The inheritance of structurally abnormal hemoglobins follows simple mendelian laws. This patient's husband also has hemoglobin E trait. There are four children. What would be the expected distribution of their hemoglobin types? (Select one.)

1. HGB A, HGB AE, HGB E
        1   :   1   :   2

[   ]

2. HGB A, HGB AE, HGB E
    1   :   2   :   1
[   ]

3. HGB A, HGB AE, HGB E
    2   :   1   :   1
[   ]

Section X

The probability, in this mating, would be to have one normal offspring, two with hemoglobin E trait, and one with homozygous hemoglobin E.

Go to the Enrichment Section.

Enrichment Section

Hemoglobin E trait is seen most commonly in Southeast Asians; however, this hemoglobin trait is not limited to this ethnic group. Hemoglobin E trait occurs once in about every 70,000 North Americans of European ancestry. Today, because of the influx of Southeast Asians into this country, hemoglobin E trait is one of the more frequently encountered hemoglobin variants in the United States.

Individuals with hemoglobin E trait usually have no anemia. Microcytosis is a feature of this hemoglobin variant and in some cases there will be erythrocytosis. Hemoglobin E trait is entirely innocuous and patients with this finding should be reassured of its benignity. The homozygous condition for hemoglobin E is also benign. Because of the microcytosis, the most common clinical problem is to distinguish hemoglobin E trait from simple iron deficiency.

Bibliography

Fairbanks VF: Hemoglobinopathies and Thalassemias: Laboratory Methods and Case Studies. New York, Brian C Decker, 1980

Hillman RS, Finch CA: Red Cell Manual, 5th ed. Philadelphia, FA Davis, 1985

Case 8

A 52-YEAR-OLD MAN was first seen with complaints of weakness, loss of libido, moderate weight loss, and palpitations that had first been noticed one year previously. The liver was firm and moderately enlarged and the patient noted that his skin had become slightly darker during the past few years. The patient consumes two alcoholic beverages every evening and takes vitamin C, 1500 mg/day.

Section A
Select as many test results as you consider helpful in pinpointing the cause of the disorder. When sufficient data have been evaluated, turn to Section H.

1. GGT
   [   ]

2. AST/ALT
   [   ]

3. ALP
   [   ]

4. HGB/HCT
   [   ]

5. Differential
   [   ]

6. RBC indices

[

]

7. Serum Fe and TIBC

[

]

8. % Saturation
[   ]

9. Serum ferritin
[   ]

10. Protein electrophoresis
[   ]

11. Urine porphyrin studies
[   ]

12. Desferrioxamine excretion test
[   ]

13. Prussian blue stain of a bone marrow aspirate
[   ]

Section B

TIBC is an indirect measure of which substance? (Select one.)

1. Ferritin
[   ]

2. Transferrin
[   ]

3. Hemosiderin
[   ]

Section C

Percent saturation is calculated by the following formula:

$$\frac{\text{Serum Fe}}{\text{TIBC}} \times 100$$

Transferrin is normally 30% saturated with iron with a range of 20% to 55%.

Return to Section A and select again.

Section D

Ferritin is the major form in which the body's storage iron is normally present. It is found in particularly high concentration in the liver, spleen, and bone marrow. Serum ferritin levels generally reflect the proportion of total iron in the body present as storage iron.

Return to Section A and select again.

Section E
The desferrioxamine excretion test determines the degree of iron overload by measuring the 24-hour urine iron excretion following intramuscular injection of desferrioxamine, an iron-chelating agent. Normal excretion is <2 mg iron/24 hr.

Return to Section A and select again.

Section F
The Prussian blue stain of a bone marrow aspirate is performed to determine the amount of iron stores in the reticuloendothelial (RE) system.

Return to Section A or go to Section H.

Section G
Transferrin is a β_1 globulin and is the major iron-transport protein. The TIBC indirectly measures the amount of transferrin by determining the total amount of iron that could be bound by transferrin when it is completely saturated with iron. Normally, transferrin is 30% saturated with iron.

Return to section A and select again.

Section H
Based on your previously collected data, select the most probable cause of this patient's symptoms. (Select one.)

1. Alcoholic cirrhosis
   [   ]
2. Dietary iron overload
   [   ]
3. Porphyria cutanea tarda
   [   ]
4. Primary hemochromatosis
   [   ]
5. Sideroblastic anemia
   [   ]

Section I

Good choice, but incorrect. Extreme elevations of ferritin and liver iron are not typical of alcoholic cirrhosis. Protein electrophoresis would be abnormal and may reveal a beta-gamma bridge.

Return to Section H and select again.

Section J

The patient history reveals that the patient is not taking any iron medication and is consuming a normal diet.

Return to Section H and select again.

Section K

Porphyria cutanea tarda may be associated with increased iron stores but not to this degree. The patient's history does not reveal the cutaneous photosensitivity characteristic of this disease. Urine porphyrin analysis should reveal elevated uroporphyrins.

Return to Section H and select again.

Section L

Very good. Primary hemochromatosis is an inherited disorder of iron metabolism. Characteristically the serum iron, % saturation, and ferritin levels are extremely elevated with a decreased TIBC.

Go to Section N.

Section M

Hematologic examination reveals no evidence of anemia or abnormal erythropoiesis, which would rule out iron loading secondary to a hematologic disorder.

Return to Section H and select again.

Section N

Select all factors that tend to lower serum iron levels. (Review each choice.)

1. Diurnal variation

   [   ]

2. Infection/inflammation/malignancy

   [   ]

3. Acute hepatitis

   [   ]

4. Acute hemorrhage

   [   ]

Section O

Iron levels are subject to significant diurnal variation. Evening values are approximately one-third lower than morning values.

Return to Section N.

Section P

Numerous infections and inflammatory and malignant disorders result in stimulation of RE cells, which then release subnormal amounts of iron to transferrin. The decreased plasma iron concentration and subsequent decrease of transferrin saturation act as the stimulus to increase the rate of iron release from RE cells until stabilization occurs.

Return to Section N.

Section Q

In acute hepatitis increased serum iron levels are present due to the release of storage iron from injured hepatic cells.

Return to Section N.

Section R

Decreased serum iron levels may be seen as a result of chronic hemorrhage. Acute hemorrhage does not lower iron levels.

Go to Section S.

Section S

Select all conditions that tend to elevate serum ferritin levels out of proportion to body iron stores. (Review each choice.)

    1. Acute hepatitis
      [   ]
    2. Malignant neoplasms
      [   ]
    3. Leukemia
      [   ]
    4. Diurnal variation
      [   ]

Section T

Serum ferritin concentrations are elevated in conditions of hepatic necrosis, either viral or drug-induced. Elevations are due, in part, to the inability of the liver to remove ferritin from plasma and to the increased release of ferritin from injured parenchymal cells.

Return to Section S.

Section U

Ferritin levels are increased in chronic pathophysiologic conditions such as cancer, inflammation, or infection and are most probably due to increased synthesis. Elevated levels should be interpreted cautiously in the presence of these underlying disorders.

Return to Section S.

Section V

Leukocytes contain high concentrations of ferritin. Levels are particularly high in acute myeloblastic and myelomonocytic leukemia.

Return to Section S.

Section W

Diurnal variation does not appear to affect ferritin levels.

Go to Section X.

Section X

Select the laboratory test that is the most definitive finding for the diagnosis of primary hemochromatosis. (Select one.)

1. Serum Fe/TIBC
   [   ]
2. Serum ferritin
   [   ]
3. Liver biopsy
   [   ]
4. Prussian blue stain of a bone marrow aspirate
   [   ]

Section Y

Measurement of serum Fe and TIBC is the most useful initial diagnostic test for hemochromatosis. Serum iron concentrations range from 175 to 275 μg/dl while TIBC is decreased to less than 300 μg/dl. However, due to the nonspecificity of the tests, typical values are not definitive.

Return to Section X and select again.

Section Z

Serum ferritin levels in hemochromatosis usually range from 1000 to 10,000 ng/ml. Elevated serum ferritin concentrations can be found that are disproportionate to iron stores in underlying conditions of infection, inflammation, and malignancy, so that elevated serum ferritin levels are not definitive for hemochromatosis.

Return to Section X and select again.

Section AA
The most specific and definitive test for hemochromatosis is a liver biopsy with evaluation of iron content and its distribution within the liver lobule. The amount of iron and its distribution help to distinguish hemochromatosis from Laennec's cirrhosis, which can present with similar serum Fe, TIBC, % saturation, and ferritin levels.

Go to Section CC.

Section BB
Iron staining of bone marrow aspirates will reveal high normal to moderately increased hemosiderin deposits in the RE cells. Due to the variability in findings, the test is not definitive for hemochromatosis.

Return to Section X and select again.

Section CC
Select all other lab tests that would be likely to be abnormal in primary hemochromatosis.

1. Glucose
   [   ]
2. Hormones
   [   ]
3. Total protein
   [   ]
4. Prothrombin time
   [   ]
5. Alpha fetoprotein
   [   ]

Section DD
Diabetes mellitus is present in up to 80% of cases of hemochromatosis. Patients are likely to have increased insulin levels with decreased insulin sensitivity as a result of impaired insulin degradation due to hepatic dysfunction. Therefore, glucose intolerance is a common finding. Other factors such as familial predisposition and pancreatic insufficiency due to iron deposition are also implicated in the development of diabetes.

Return to Section CC and select again.

Section EE
As many as two-thirds of cases of hemochromatosis experience pituitary insufficiency with the primary manifestation of hypogonadism. With pituitary insufficiency, gonadotropin levels are usually decreased.

Return to Section CC and select again.

Section FF

Total protein levels are usually within the normal reference range. Minor changes in protein patterns may be seen that reflect the degree of liver impairment due to underlying cirrhosis.

Return to Section CC and select again.

Section GG

Hypoprothrombinemia may occur in hemochromatosis with advanced cirrhosis due to impairment of synthesis of coagulation factors.

Return to Section CC and select again.

Section HH

Hepatocellular carcinoma develops in approximately 15% of cases of hemochromatosis. Alpha-fetoprotein is an oncofetal antigen that is elevated in a high percentage of patients with hepatocellular carcinoma.

Go to the Enrichment Section.

Enrichment Section

Hemochromatosis refers to a group of disorders characterized by excessive iron absorption. Primary hemochromatosis is an inherited inborn error of iron metabolism. HLA typing has added to the understanding of its inheritance. In most cases there is a strong association of the disorder with HLA-A3, indicating its genetic association. It is inherited as an autosomal recessive trait.

Secondary hemochromatosis refers to a variety of disorders in which iron overload is a characteristic finding but is unrelated to a genetic disorder of iron absorption. Secondary hemochromatosis includes iron overload due to alcoholic cirrhosis, iron-loading anemias, dietary iron overload, and porphyria cutanea tarda.

In primary hemochromatosis, iron absorption through the gastrointestinal tract occurs at an excessive rate that is independent of the iron needs of the body. Normally, absorbed iron is incorporated into hemoglobin, myoglobin, and other heme-containing proteins. However, in primary hemochromatosis, excessive iron is stored in tissues of the body in the form of ferritin and hemosiderin. Eventually this excessive iron deposition leads to parenchymal cell damage and functional failure of the organs. Involved organs include primarily the liver, pancreas, and heart. Because the process of excess iron absorption and tissue deposition occurs over many years, symptoms are usually not manifest until the ages of 40 to 60 years, with a male predominance of 10:1.

The clinical manifestations depend on the type of organ involvement, but in general the disease is characterized by a triad of symptoms involving cirrhosis, diabetes, and skin pigmentation due to melanin deposition.

The frequency of other endocrine disorders such as hypothalmic or pituitary failure is variable as is the occurrence of arthropathy and cardiac disease.

The major problem in the differential diagnosis of hemochromatosis is the differentiation from alcoholic cirrhosis. Iron overload in alcoholic cirrhosis is due, in part, to increased iron absorption as a result of ineffective erythropoiesis from nutritional deficiencies and to the absorption-enhancing properties of alcohol consumption.

The combined measurements of the following parameters provide the best laboratory screening regimen for the detection of hemochromatosis:

Serum Fe   > 200 μg/dl
TIBC   < 300 μg/dl
% Saturation > 75%
Ferritin   > 1000 ng/ml

The degree of iron overload in alcoholic cirrhosis usually does not reveal the extreme elevations seen in hemochromatosis. Additionally, in alcoholic cirrhosis there is evidence of greater liver function impairment as manifest by higher enzyme elevations, jaundice, ascites, and portal hypertension.

The hematologic findings in hemochromatosis are relatively normal. Occasionally, a mild leukopenia and thrombocytopenia due to hypersplenism may be manifest. Anemia may be a prominent feature in secondary forms of iron overload, which helps distinguish these conditions from primary hemochromatosis.

Bibliography
Marchand A, Galen RS: Ironing out the problem of hemochromatosis. Diagn Med 4(3):79–81, 1981
McLaren GD, Muir WA, Kellermeyer RW: Iron overload disorders: Natural history, pathogenesis, diagnosis, and therapy. CRC Crit Rev Clin Lab Sci 19(3):205–259, 1983
Pollycove M: Hemochromatosis. In Stanbury JB, Wyngaarden JB, Frederickson DS (eds): The Metabolic Basis of Inherited Disease. New York, McGraw-Hill, 1978

Case 9

A 57-YEAR-OLD MAN was admitted to the hospital because of suspected kidney stone. Symptoms had begun six months earlier. The symptoms included abdominal and back pain, easy fatigability, myalgia, and constipation.

The patient's admission work-up included the following results:

Total protein	=	6.2 g/dl
Albumin	=	3.3 g/dl
Calcium	=	14.0 mg/dl
Phosphorus	=	1.5 mg/dl
Alkaline phosphatase (ALP)	=	315 U/l
Lactic dehydrogenase (LD)	=	125 U/l

Which of these results would be considered abnormal? (Select as many as appropriate.)

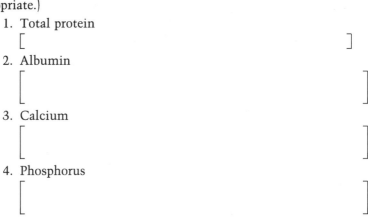

1. Total protein
   [   ]
2. Albumin
   [   ]
3. Calcium
   [   ]
4. Phosphorus
   [   ]

5. ALP

$$\left[\qquad\qquad\qquad\qquad\qquad \right]$$

6. LD

$$\left[\qquad\qquad\qquad\qquad\qquad \right]$$

Section A

Before interpreting a calcium level, which of the following calculations should be performed? (Select one.)

1. Measured serum calcium—serum albumin + 4.0

$$\left[\qquad\qquad\qquad\qquad\qquad \right]$$

2. $1.86 \times \text{sodium} + \dfrac{\text{glucose}}{18} + \dfrac{\text{BUN}}{2.8}$

$$\left[\qquad\qquad\qquad\qquad\qquad \right]$$

3. $\dfrac{\text{Measured calcium}}{0.6 + (\text{total protein}/19.4)}$

$$\left[\qquad\qquad\qquad\qquad\qquad \right]$$

4. $\dfrac{(98 - 0.8) \times (\text{age} - 20)}{\text{Serum creatinine}}$

$$\left[\qquad\qquad\qquad\qquad\qquad \right]$$

Section B

Select the most common cause of hypercalcemia. (Select one.)

1. Secondary hyperparathyroidism

$$\left[\qquad\qquad\qquad\qquad\qquad \right]$$

2. Malignancy

$$\left[\qquad\qquad\qquad\qquad\qquad \right]$$

3. Hyperthyroidism

$$\left[\qquad\qquad\qquad\qquad\qquad \right]$$

4. Primary hyperparathyroidism

[

]

5. Multiple myeloma

[

]

Section C

Select the most common cause leading to primary hyperparathyroidism. (Select one.)

1. Parathyroid adenoma

[

]

2. Parathyroid hyperplasia

[

]

3. Carcinoma of the parathyroid

[

]

Section D

Parathyroid hormone (PTH) is produced in the chief ("water-clear") cells in the parathyroid glands. Which of the following mechanisms does this hormone use to produce its biological action? (Select one.)

1. Mobile receptor model

[   ]

2. Fixed receptor model

[   ]

Section E

Most of the steroid hormones utilize the mobile receptor model to produce their biological actions. The steroid hormones circulate attached to a specific protein. The steroid is released from the carrier protein and traverses the cell membrane where it then attaches to another steroid receptor protein. This steroid–receptor complex binds to a nuclear acceptor where it causes gene activation or derepression and subsequently stimulates the production of messenger RNA and protein synthesis.

Go back to Section D and select again.

Section F

The biological action of parathyroid hormone (PTH) like that of other polypeptide hormones, is to stimulate adenyl cyclase in the target tissues. The peptide hormones circulate in a free state and then attach to a specific receptor on the cell wall. This combination activates the cell-membrane–bound adenyl cyclase, which catalyzes the conversion of ATP to cyclic AMP (cAMP). Cyclic AMP activates a protein kinase that in turn converts an inactive enzyme to an active enzyme.

Go to Section G.

Section G

PTH is synthesized in the parathyroid glands as a prohormone. The prohormone is converted to the storage form, which is secreted into the blood. In the liver and kidneys, PTH is cleaved into at least two major fragments. The N-terminal fragment has the physiological activity, whereas the C-terminal fragment has no physiological activity. Of the following PTH assays currently available, which is considered to be the most specific for primary hyperparathyroidism? (Select one.)

1. Intact PTH

2. C-terminal PTH

3. N-terminal PTH

Section H

The main function of PTH is to regulate the concentration of free calcium. PTH does this by its effects on bone, on kidney, and, indirectly, on the small intestine. Select the physiological effect that PTH has on the bone. (Select as many as appropriate.)

1. Causes bone resorption and bone formation

2. Increases bone cell activity

$$\Big[\Big]$$

3. Decreases bone cell activity

$$[]$$

4. Increases bone cell mass

$$[]$$

Section I

Select the physiological effect of PTH on the kidneys. (Select three.)

1. Enhances the renal tubular absorption of phosphate

$$[]$$

2. Inhibits the renal tubular absorption of phosphate

$$\Big[\Big]$$

3. Increases reabsorption of free calcium in the distal tubule

$$\Big[\Big]$$

4. Decreases reabsorption of free calcium in the distal tubule

$$[]$$

5. Enhances the absorption of bicarbonate (HCO_3^-) and enhances the exchange of tubular hydrogen ions (H^+) for luminal sodium ions (Na^+)

$$[]$$

6. Inhibits the absorption of HCO_3^- and inhibits the exchange of tubular H^+ for luminal Na^+

$$\Big[\Big]$$

Section J

The tubular reabsorption of phosphorus (TRP) can be calculated after concentrations of phosphorus (P) and creatinine (Cr) have been determined on a fasting serum sample and first morning urine sample. Select the correct formula for TRP.

1. $\text{TRP} (\%) = 1 - \dfrac{\text{Serum P}}{\text{Urine P}} \times \dfrac{\text{Serum Cr}}{\text{Urine Cr}} \times 100$

$$[]$$

2. $\text{TRP}(\%) = 1 + \dfrac{\text{Serum P}}{\text{Serum Cr}} \times \dfrac{\text{Urine P}}{\text{Urine Cr}} \times 100$

[   ]

3. $\text{TRP}(\%) = 1 - \dfrac{\text{Urine P}}{\text{Serum P}} \times \dfrac{\text{Serum Cr}}{\text{Urine Cr}} \times 100$

[   ]

Section K

PTH causes an indirect effect on the small intestine by doing which of the following? (Select one.)

1. Inhibits the conversion of 25-hydroxy cholecalciferol to 1,25-dihydroxy cholecalciferol

   [   ]

2. Enhances the conversion of 25-hydroxy cholecalciferol to 1,25-dihydroxy cholecalciferol

   [   ]

3. Enhances the conversion of 7-dehydrocholesterol to cholecalciferol

   [   ]

Section L

Many organs and tissues are affected in primary hyperparathyroidism. Review each of the following organs or tissues that may be affected.

1. Bone

   [   ]

2. Kidneys

   [   ]

3. Pancreas

   [   ]

4. Gastrointestinal tract

   [   ]

Continued

5. Cardiovascular system

6. Central nervous system

7. Soft tissues

Section M

Some patients have only minimal bone changes while others may manifest bone cysts, "brown tumors," or osteitis fibrosa cystica. Bone cysts may occur when there is focally excessive resorption of the bone. "Brown tumors" are focal hemorrhagic lesions that occur because of hemorrhage in the focal areas where structural support of the bone is lost when resorption is excessive. Generalized osteitis fibrosa cystica consists of a profound evidence of bone resorption with bone cysts, excessive osteoclastic activity, and secondary fibrosis. Because of the effect of the PTH, the osteoclasts cause resorption of bone with a diminished bone mass. Later in the course of the disease, the osteoblasts will increase in number and lay down uncalcified osteoid. Osteitis fibrosa cystica is also known as which of the following? (Select one.)

1. Osteomalacia

2. Osteoporosis

3. Osteopetrosis

4. von Recklinghausen's disease

Section N

From the following list of laboratory findings, select those that would be abnormal in primary hyperparathyroidism:

1. Serum calcium increased

    [   ]

2. Serum calcium decreased

    [   ]

3. Serum phosphorus increased

    [   ]

4. Serum phosphorus decreased

    [   ]

5. Urine calcium increased

    [   ]

6. Urine calcium decreased

    [   ]

7. Urine phosphorus increased

    [   ]

8. Urine phosphorus decreased

    [   ]

9. Serum alkaline phosphatase increased

    [   ]

10. Serum alkaline phosphatase decreased

    [   ]

11. Urine hydroxyproline increased

    [

Continued

12. Urine hydroxyproline decreased
    [   ]
13. Urine cAMP increased
    [   ]
14. Urine cAMP decreased
    [   ]
15. Serum chloride increased
    [   ]
16. Serum chloride decreased
    [   ]
17. Serum bicarbonate increased.
    [   ]
18. Serum bicarbonate decreased
    [

    ]
19. Blood pH increased
    [   ]
20. Blood pH decreased
    [   ]

Section O

Urinary adenosine 3′,5′-cyclic monophosphate (cAMP) is useful in differentiating primary hyperparathyroidism from other causes of hypercalcemia. PTH activates adenyl cyclase in the kidney, which increases the cAMP concentration. The increased levels of cAMP stimulate the renal enzyme that converts 25-hydroxy cholecalciferol to 1,25-dihydroxy cholecalciferol, which in turn causes increased absorption of calcium from the small intestine.

The cAMP found in the urine is derived from two sources: (1) that derived by glomerular filtration of plasma, and (2) that synthesized in the kidney and excreted by the renal tubular cells. Increased levels of urinary cAMP are observed in primary hyperparathyroidism and decreased levels are found in patients with nonparathyroid hypercalcemia, hypoparathyroidism, and pseudohypoparathyroidism. However, a normal or increased urinary cAMP concentration does not differentiate between hyperparathyroidism, ectopic secretion of PTH by a tumor, or the hypercalcemia of malignancy. As a matter of fact, the urinary cAMP may be elevated in cancer patients who have a normal serum calcium level. The reason for the increased urinary cAMP levels in these patients remains unexplained.

Go back to Section N and select again or go to Section Q.

Section P

PTH acts on the renal tubular cells and inhibits the reabsorption of bicarbonate and the exchange of tubular H^+ for luminal Na^+. Which type of acid–base imbalance is exhibited by patients with primary hyperparathyroidism? (Select one.)

    1. Metabolic alkalosis

    2. Respiratory alkalosis

    3. Metabolic acidosis

    4. Respiratory acidosis

Section Q

From the following list, select the treatment of primary hyperparathyroidism. (Review each choice.)

    1. Surgical management

    2. Medical management

Section R

Hyperparathyroidism is a prominent feature of several syndromes involving polyglandular adenomas or hyperplasia. These syndromes are familial and are called *multiple endocrine adenomas* (MEA). Identify the other gland abnormalities found in MEA type I. (Select as many as appropriate.)

1. Pituitary

[
]

2. Thyroid

[
]

3. Adrenal medulla

[   ]

4. Adrenal cortex

[
]

5. Pancreas

[
]

Section S

Hyperparathyroidism may also be associated with MEA type II, which is inherited as an autosomal dominant trait. Identify the other gland abnormalities found in MEA type II. (Select as many as appropriate.)

1. Pituitary

[   ]

2. Thyroid

[
]

3. Adrenal medulla

[
]

4. Adrenal cortex

[   ]

5. Pancreas

[   ]

Enrichment Section

The parathyroid glands secrete parathyroid hormone (PTH), which is concerned with maintaining a normal plasma calcium level. Hyperparathyroidism is the cause in 10% to 30% of the hypercalcemic patients. The incidence of hyperparathyroidism ranges from 1 in 400 to 1 in 1000. The peak incidence is around the sixth decade and the female-to-male ratio is approximately 1.6 : 1.

Primary hyperparathyroidism may be caused by single or multiple benign adenomas, carcinoma, or hyperplasia. Regardless of the cause, there is eventually an excessive secretion of PTH. The PTH causes an enhanced intestinal calcium absorption from the small intestine, an increased bone resorption, and an increased renal calcium retention.

The most common manifestations of primary hyperparathyroidism are kidney and bone disorders. The hypercalcemia and hypercalciuria lead to an impaired ability of the kidney to concentrate urine; polyuria and nocturia may result. Nephrolithiasis is a very common complication. Nephrocalcinosis may produce a variety of tubular defects, including amino aciduria and renal tubular acidosis.

About 15% of patients with primary hyperparathyroidism have symptomatic bone disease. Osteitis fibrosa cystica is the classic bone disease of hyperparathyroidism.

The treatment of choice remains surgery with the extirpation of the tumor(s) that is present in 75% to 80% of the cases. Subtotal parathyroidectomy with autotransplantation is recommended in patients with diffuse granular hyperplasia.

Bibliography

Bakerman S, Prabakher K: Calcium metabolism and hypercalcemia. Lab Manag 20:17–25, 1982

Hall R, Evered D, Greene R: Color Atlas of Endocrinology. Chicago, Year Book Medical Publishers, 1979

Hershman JM: Endocrine Pathophysiology: A Patient-Oriented Approach, 2nd ed. Philadelphia, Lea & Febiger, 1982

Hershman JM: Practical Endocrinology. New York, Wiley Medical Publication, 1981

Kubasik NP: Cyclic AMP. Clin Chem News 10:21, 1984

Lindall AW: New tests diagnose mineral disease. Clin Chem News 9:14, 1983

Mallette LE et al: Evaluation of hypocalcemia with a highly sensitive, homologous radioimmunoassay for the midregion of parathyroid hormone. Pediatrics 71:64–69, 1983

Mazzaferri EL: Endocrinology, 2nd ed. New York, Medical Examination Publishing, 1980

Recker RR, Saville PD: Hypercalcemia and hypocalcemia in clinical practice. Hosp Med 15:74–90, 1979

Zawada ET: Diagnosis: Causes of hypercalcemia. Hosp Med 17:94–102, 1981

Case 10

A 20-MONTH-OLD BLACK GIRL, without previous medical history, was taken to the emergency room after a 12-hour period of irritability and abdominal pain with some symptoms of upper respiratory infection. There was no vomiting or diarrhea, only an occasional cough. The patient's temperature was 100.5° F; pulse 155; respirations 44; blood pressure 110/60; weight 29 pounds, 5 ounces. The physical examination was remarkable only for abdominal tenderness in the right upper and lower quadrants. No spleen was palpable. Initial radiology and laboratory data were as follows:

Chest and abdominal x-rays were essentially normal.
Chemistries

Blood urea nitrogen	=	10 mg/dl
Sodium	=	136 mmol/l
Potassium	=	4.3 mmol/l
Chloride	=	99 mmol/l
CO_2	=	21 mmol/l

Go to Section A.

Section A
Which of the chemistry results are abnormal? (Review all choices.)

1. Blood urea nitrogen (BUN)
[   ]

2. Sodium, potassium, chloride
[   ]

3. CO_2
[   ]

Section B
In children and adults, the BUN reference range is 5 to 20 mg/dl.

Return to Section A.

Section C
In children and adults, the reference ranges are as follows: Na = 136 to 146 mmol/l; K = 3.5 to 5.1 mmol/l; and Cl = 98 to 106 mmol/l.

Return to Section A.

Section D
The CO_2 reference range in children is 18 to 27 mmol/l.

Go to Section E.

Section E
The urinalysis showed a specific gravity of 1.018, 1+ ketones, and an essentially negative microscopic result. Why might this patient have 1+ ketones? (Select one.)

1. The Na and K levels suggest a reason for 1+ ketones.

   [   ]

2. The presence of fever is associated with ketonuria.

   [   ]

3. The CO_2 level suggests that there could be a correlated increase in urinary ketones.

   [   ]

Section F
Ketonuria often accompanies the restricted carbohydrate intake that occurs in association with fever.

Go to Section G.

Section G
The CBC and reticulocyte count were as follows:

WBC   = $11.1 \times 10^3/\mu l$
RBC   = $4.05 \times 10^6/\mu l$
HGB   = 11.2 g/dl
HCT   = 32%
MCV   = 79 fl
MCH   = 27.7 pg
MCHC   = 35.0 g/dl
Reticulocyte
  count   = 2.1%

Which of these hematological data are abnormal? (Review all choices.)

1. WBC

   [   ]

2. RBC, HGB, HCT

   [   ]

3. MCV, MCH, MCHC
[   ]
4. Reticulocyte count
[   ]

Section H

The WBC count is slightly elevated. The reference range is 4.0 to 10.0 × $10^3/\mu l$.

Return to Section G.

Section I

The RBC, HGB, and HCT are borderline low. The mean RBC value for this age is 4.7 × $10^6/\mu l$ and the HGB and HCT reference ranges are 10.5 to 13.5 g/dl and 33% to 39%, respectively.

Return to Section G.

Section J

The MCV, MCH, and MCHC are normal. The MCV and MCH reference ranges, in children 18 months to 4 years, are 74 to 86 fl and 24 to 30 pg, respectively; the MCHC in children and adults is 31 to 35 g/dl.

Return to Section G.

Section K

The reticulocyte count is slightly elevated. The reference range in children and adults is 0.5% to 1.5%.

Go to Section L.

Section L

The differential and blood smear evaluation were as follows:

75% neutrophils
10% bands
13% lymphocytes
 2% monocytes
WBC morphology
    Normal
Platelets
    Adequate
RBC morphology
    Target cells
    Anisocytosis
    Slight polychromasia

The patient was admitted to the pediatric ward for further observation. Her abdominal examination gradually normalized over the next two days; however, she remained febrile to 101.8°F through the third hospital day. At that time, throat, blood, and urine cultures were all negative for organisms. The hematocrit and reticulocyte counts remained stable.

In review of this patient's data, is there anything significant that would suggest further investigation? (Select one.)

1. No
   [   ]
2. Yes
   [   ]

Section M
The finding of target cells, anisocytosis, and polychromasia on the peripheral blood smear was significant and a hemoglobin electrophoresis (pH 8.6) was ordered. What would be the expected results in this patient? (Select one.)

1. HGB A, S, A_2 increased
   [   ]
2. HGB A, F increased; A_2 decreased
   [   ]
3. HGB A, C
   [   ]
4. HGB S, C
   [   ]

Section N
Two major hemoglobin bands, with hemoglobin A comprising 58% of the total hemoglobin and hemoglobin S comprising 38% of the total hemoglobin, were found in a case representing Section M, 1. There was 3.5% hemoglobin A_2. The solubility test for hemoglobin S was positive. The patient wasn't anemic, the reticulocyte count was 1.0%, and the red blood cell indices and the blood smear were normal. These findings are typical of hemoglobin S trait, a hemoglobinopathy found in approximately 8% of American blacks.

Go back to Section M and select another alternative.

Section O
Hemoglobin A was quantified at 17%, hemoglobin F at 82%, and hemoglobin A_2 at less than 1% in a case representing Section M, 2. This 3-day-old black patient had a normal hematocrit for her age, a reticulocyte count of 2.8%, and macrocytic red blood cell indices. There were polychromatophi-

lic red cells on the blood smear. These results are normal in the early newborn period.

Go back to Section M and select another alternative.

Section P
The patient in a case representing Section M, 3, had normal red blood cell indices, no anemia, a normal reticulocyte count, and target cells on the blood smear. The patient was asymptomatic. Hemoglobin A was quantified at 60% and hemoglobin C (+A$_2$) at 40%. Hemoglobin C was confirmed by agar gel electrophoresis. These findings are typical of hemoglobin C trait, a hemoglobin abnormality occurring in approximately 3% of American blacks.

Go back to Section M and select another alternative.

Section Q
Two slow-moving electrophoretic bands were quantified at 57% hemoglobin S and 43% hemoglobin C (+A$_2$). These were confirmed by citrate agar electrophoresis, which revealed bands in the S and C positions. The electrophoretic results in Section M, 4, represent hemoglobin SC disease—the diagnosis made in this case.

Go to Section R.

Section R
If a solubility test for hemoglobin S had been done in this case, what would be the expected result? (Select one.)

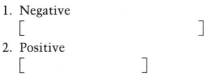

    1. Negative
       [   ]
    2. Positive
       [   ]

Section S
A positive solubility test is presumptive evidence for hemoglobin S. However, every positive solubility test should be confirmed by hemoglobin electrophoresis since rare sickling hemoglobins such as C$_{Georgetown}$ will also give a positive result.

Go to Section T.

Section T
The patient's temperature was 99.2°F on the fourth hospital day and had returned to normal within 24 hours. The patient was discharged.

    One month later, this 21-month-old with known SC disease returned to the pediatric ward with the complaint of an inability to bear weight on the right knee. There was no history of trauma to the knee or a previous painful joint. The patient was admitted for observation. Her oral temperature was 100°F. The routine urinalysis examination was negative. A WBC, HGB, HCT, differential, and smear evaluation were ordered with the following results:

WBC = 10.3 × 10³/μl
HGB = 12.0 g/dl
HCT = 33%
Differential
        75% neutrophils
        2% bands
        21% lymphocytes
        2% monocytes
WBC morphology
        Normal
Platelets
        Adequate
RBC morphology
        Target cells
        Polychromasia
        Few red blood cell fragments

A serum alkaline phosphatase was ordered. What result would be expected in this case? (Select one.)

        1. 150 U/l
            [   ]
        2. 390 U/l
            [   ]

Section U
The alkaline phosphatase reference range in a female <10 years is 120 to 310 U/l, and 150 U/l was not the result obtained.

Go back to Section T.

Section V
An elevated alkaline phosphatase often accompanies SC disease, >310 U/l for this age.

Go to Section W.

Section W
Careful examination failed to reveal any otitis, evidence of pneumonia or meningitis, or evidence of urinary tract infection. The child was observed for 48 hours and during this period she regained function of the knee. Her temperature returned to normal and she was dismissed to be followed

routinely by her physician. At this time her temperature spikes were thought to be secondary to her disease.

Go to the Enrichment Section.

Enrichment Section

The most frequent sickling disorder after sickle cell anemia (~1 : 400 blacks at birth) is hemoglobin SC disease. This syndrome tends to run a milder course than sickle cell anemia and is associated with less frequent crises and a much less severe hemolytic anemia.

Hemoglobin SC disease is estimated to occur in approximately 1 of every 800 births among American blacks. It is important because of the occurrence of serious vaso-occlusive complications. These include eye lesions characterized by vitreous hemorrhages and retinitis proliferans occasionally proceeding to retinal detachment and blindness. Other complications are surprisingly frequent and include joint and abdominal pain, hematuria, epistaxis, and concomitant infections. Hematuria, vitreous hemorrhages, and splenomegaly typically are complications of adult life. The frequency of extremity pain in youth and its tendency to decrease with age may be related to the increased metabolism and relatively inadequate blood supply of rapidly growing tissue.

This case represents some typical findings in hemoglobin SC disease. Often there is bizarre abdominal pain, usually of obscure origin, and muscle, bone, and joint pain. Pulmonary symptoms include chest pain, fever, and cough, together with a leukocytosis. The high incidence of pulmonary disease is probably due to factors favoring sickling in the pulmonary vasculature. The alkaline phosphatase is frequently elevated, a finding that is related to bone disease rather than liver dysfunction. In the absence of a second disease process, patients with SC disease are usually not severely anemic. It is important to stress, however, that during periods of illness, anemia may become significant. Polychromatophilia is present in most blood films, reflecting accelerated erythropoiesis and probably marrow damage due to microinfarcts of the marrow. Anisocytosis and targeting are characteristic of this syndrome. Sickle cells may or may not be seen.

Hemoglobin SC disease is an inherited disorder in which the gene for S hemoglobin is inherited from one parent and the gene for C hemoglobin from the other. This genetic constellation is designated as a doubly heterozygous state. Although a number of clinical and hematological features suggest SC disease, the diagnosis must be based on results from tests such as the electrophoretic studies of hemoglobin.

Bibliography

Fairbanks VF: Hemoglobinopathies and Thalassemias: Laboratory Methods and Case Studies. New York, Brian C Decker, 1980

Lichtman MA: Hematology and Oncology. New York, Grune & Stratton, 1980

Case 11

A 29-YEAR-OLD WOMAN was admitted to the emergency room with acute abdominal pain that had persisted for the past three days, accompanied by headache, constipation, hypertension, tachycardia, nausea, and vomiting. She had previously suffered from periods of depression and hysterical behavior and was diagnosed as schizophrenic. She was released from the psychiatric services of a hospital two years previously. Select all laboratory tests that you would like to evaluate at this time:

1. AST/ALT
[   ]

2. ALP
[   ]

3. Amylase
[   ]

4. Glucose
[   ]

5. Electrolytes
[

]

6. WBC
[   ]

7. RBC
[   ]

8. HGB/HCT
[
]

9. Differential

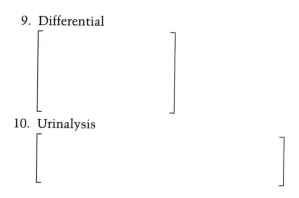

10. Urinalysis

Section A

Select any additional tests that would be significant in pinpointing the disorder.

1. T_3 and T_4

    [   ]

2. ADH

    [   ]

3. Watson-Schwartz test

    [   ]

4. Trace metal screen

    [   ]

5. Drug screen

    [   ]

Go to Section B.

Section B

Based on your accumulated data, select the condition that best correlates with those data:

1. Thyrotoxicosis

    [   ]

2. Syndrome of inappropriate ADH secretion

    [   ]

3. Porphyria

    [   ]

4. Trace metal toxicity

    [   ]

5. Drug toxicity

    [   ]

Section C

Increased levels of ADH leading to SIADH are secondary to the pathophysiologic condition and not the primary cause of this patient's symptoms.
Increased ADH levels contribute to the observed electrolyte abnormalities. Other laboratory findings are not consistent with a primary condition
of SIADH.

Return to Section C and select again.

Section D

The Watson-Schwartz test is a screening test for the presence of porphobilinogen in the urine. A positive test is preliminary evidence for one of the
inherited porphyrias.

Go to Section G.

Section E

Trace metal toxicity, especially lead poisoning, could account for this
patient's neurological symptoms and acute abdominal pain, but all tests
are negative, ruling out lead poisoning or other trace metal toxicity. The
Watson-Schwartz test is negative in lead poisoning.

Return to Section B and select again.

Section F

A drug overdose could account for this patient's neurological symptoms
and acute abdominal pain but all tests are negative, ruling out drug toxicity.

Return to Section B and select again.

Section G

The Watson-Schwartz test utilizes Ehrlich's reagent (p-dimethylamino-
benzaldehyde), which is not specific for porphobilinogen (PBG) and will
give a positive reaction with other substances. Select the most common
interfering substance that will give a positive Watson-Schwartz reaction.

1. d-Amino levulinic acid
   [   ]

2. Bilirubin
   [   ]

3. Urobilinogen
   [

   ]

4. 5-HIAA
   [   ]

Section H

Because of the potential for a false positive Watson-Schwartz test, PBG and
UBG should be separated. Separation is based on differential solubility
using chloroform and butanol. Select the correct solubility characteristic
of PBG.

　　1. Soluble in chloroform
　　　[　　　　　　　　　　　　　　]
　　2. Soluble in butanol
　　　[　　　　　　　　　　　　　　]
　　3. Soluble in chloroform and butanol
　　　[　　　　　　　]
　　4. Insoluble in chloroform and butanol

　　　[　　　　　　　　　　　　　　　　　　　　　]

Section I

At this point, based on the clinical symptoms and a positive Watson-
Schwartz test, you suspect the patient has some type of porphyria. Select
the next laboratory test to be performed in this patient's work-up.

　　1. RBC enzyme studies
　　　[　　　　　　　]
　　2. Fecal porphyrin analysis
　　　[　　　　　　　]
　　3. Erythrocyte porphyrin analysis
　　　[　　　　　　　]
　　4. Quantitative PBG/urine porphyrin analysis
　　　[　　　　　　　]
　　5. d-ALA
　　　[　　　　　　　]

Section J

A positive Watson-Schwartz test should be confirmed by a quantitative
analysis of PBG levels to evaluate potential false positive results. Total
urine porphyrin levels are frequently done in conjunction with quantitative PBG, although in this patient total urine porphyrin levels reveal little
additional diagnostic information.

Go to Section K.

Section K

The clinical symptoms in addition to laboratory data are important in
aiding in the differential diagnosis of the porphyrias. Select the major
categories of clinical symptoms. (Review all choices.)

1. Cutaneous photosensitivity
   [   ]
2. Neurological disturbances
   [   ]
3. Hemolytic anemia
   [   ]
4. Gastrointestinal disturbances
   [   ]

Section L

Cutaneous photosensitivity is one of the two main categories of clinical symptoms typical in certain types of porphyrias. It is manifested by lesions on exposed parts of the skin ranging from mild to severe with scarring and deformity. The photosensitive lesions are most likely caused by oxidative injury to the lysosomal membrane of the skin by singlet oxygen produced by accumulated porphyrins that have absorbed electromagnetic radiation in the 400-nm band.

Return to Section K and select again.

Section M

Neurological symptoms constitute one of the two main categories of clinical symptoms that occur only in those porphyrias associated with excess production of the porphyrin precursors ALA and PBG. Neurological manifestations include abnormal behavior, delirium, and seizures. Some types of porphyria can exhibit both cutaneous photosensitivity and neurological symptoms simultaneously.

Return to Section K and select again.

Section N

Hemolytic anemia occurs rarely in those porphyrias where the predominant biochemical abnormality is manifest in the erythropoietic system.

Return to Section K and select again.

Section O

Gastrointestinal symptoms commonly occur in conjunction with neurological manifestations and therefore are not considered as a separate category for classification of the porphyrias. The most common gastrointestinal symptoms are abdominal pain, vomiting, and constipation.

Go to Section P.

Section P

The patient in this case presents with an acute attack of neurological and gastrointestinal symptoms but an absence of cutaneous photosensitivity.

The initial screening test for a suspected porphyria in this category is the Watson-Schwartz test for PBG. On the basis of the clinical symptoms and positive qualitative and quantitative tests for PBG, the next laboratory test to be performed to differentiate the type of porphyria should be: (Review each choice.)

     1. RBC enzyme studies
     [   ]
     2. Fecal porphyrin analysis
     [   ]
     3. Erythrocyte porphyrin analysis
     [   ]
     4. d-ALA
     [   ]

Section Q

Identification of a specific enzyme deficiency would establish the type of porphyria. However, RBC enzyme tests are not routinely available in the clinical lab and there is some overlap in the range of levels for normal and affected individuals, making interpretation difficult at times. This case shows decreased activity of uroporphyrinogen I synthetase.

Return to Section P and select again.

Section R

The type of porphyria can usually be differentiated based on the separation and identification of fecal porphyrins in patients exhibiting these symptoms and elevated PBG levels. This patient has normal fecal porphyrin levels.

Go to Section U.

Section S

Erythrocyte porphyrin levels are not helpful in differentiating this group of porphyrias. All porphyrias in this group have normal erythrocyte porphyrin levels.

Return to Section P and select again.

Section T

d-ALA levels are commonly increased in this group of porphyrias as well as other pathophysiological conditions. It is a nonspecific test and is not helpful in differentiating this group of porphyrias.

Return to Section P and select again.

Table 1   Significant Biochemical Findings

	EP**	PBG	Total Urine Porphyrin	Fecal Copro	Proto	Neurological Signs	Skin Lesions
CEP	↑	N	↑*	↑	N	—	+
EP	↑↑*	N	N	N	↑	—	+
AIP	N	↑↑*	↑	N	N	+	—
HC	N	↑	↑	↑↑*	↑	+	—/(+)
VP	N	↑	↑	↑	↑↑*	+/(—)	—/(+)
PCT	N	N	↑↑*	↑	N	—	+

* Most significant biochemical finding

** Erythrocyte protoporphyrin

CEP, congenital erythropoietic porphyria; EP, erythropoietic protoporphyria; AIP, acute intermittent porphyria; HC, hereditary coproporphyria; VP, variegate porphyria; PCT, porphyria cutanea tarda.

Section U

Table 1 is a summary of the diagnostic biochemical findings of the porphyrias. Based on the patient's history and the accumulated laboratory data, select the most probable type of porphyria.

1. Congenital erythropoietic porphyria
   [   ]

2. Erythropoietic protoporphyria
   [   ]

3. Acute intermittent porphyria
   [   ]

4. Hereditary coproporphyria
   [   ]

5. Variegate porphyria
   [   ]

6. Porphyria cutanea tarda
   [   ]

Section V

In congenital erythropoietic porphyria, d-ALA and PBG are typically normal. Significant increases are found in both erythrocyte and urine porphyrins. The clinical symptoms are characterized by severe cutaneous photosensitivity with scarring and deformity and the absence of neurological symptoms.

Return to Section U and select again.

Section W

No biochemical abnormalities are present in the urine in erythrocyte protoporphyria. The most diagnostic finding is elevated erythrocyte protoporphyrin. The clinical symptoms are characterized by cutaneous photosensitivity and the absence of neurological symptoms.

Return to Section U and select again.

Section X

Correct. The cause of acute intermittent porphyria is a deficiency of uroporphyrinogen I synthetase with a resultant increase in urine porphyrins and porphyrin precursors.

Go to the Enrichment Section.

Section Y

Good choice, but incorrect. The urine porphyrin and PBG results are similar to these but the most diagnostic finding is elevated fecal porphyrin with a predominance of coproporphyrin. Cutaneous lesions occur rarely.

Return to Section U and select again.

Section Z

In addition to elevated porphyrin precursors and urine porphyrins, increased fecal porphyrins are found with a predominance of protoporphyrin. Cutaneous symptoms accompany neurological symptoms in approximately 50% of cases.

Return to Section U and select again.

Section AA

d-ALA and PBG are typically normal in porphyria cutanea tarda with increases of urine and fecal porphyrins. Photosensitivity is the major symptom with absence of neurological signs.

Return to Section U and select again.

Enrichment Section

Porphyrinogens are colorless compounds that consist of four pyrrole rings linked by methene bridges. The porphyrinogens are direct intermediates in the biosynthetic pathway of heme. In contrast, porphyrins are fluorescent compounds derived as by-products through oxidation of the porphyrinogens. The structures of the porphyrinogens differ according to the types of side chains attached to the pyrrole ring. The variation in side chains confers differing solubility properties on the porphyrins. Uroporphyrinogen with eight carboxyl groups is water-soluble and excreted primarily in the urine as uroporphyrin. Successive decarboxylation steps reduce coproporphyrinogen to four carboxyl groups and protoporphyrinogen to two. Thus, protoporphyrinogen is less water-soluble and is excreted almost entirely in the feces. Coproporphyrinogen is intermediate and can be excreted by either route but is preferentially excreted in the feces. The porphyrin precursors ALA and PBG are excreted almost entirely in the urine.

Each step in the biosynthesis of heme is catalyzed by a specific enzymatic reaction. Table 2 outlines the steps of the heme biosynthetic pathway. The porphyrias are disorders that result from the genetic deficiency of one of these specific enzymes, resulting in the excretion of various porphyrins, porphyrinogens, and/or porphyrin precursors in the urine and/or feces.

One useful classification of the porphyrias is to categorize them according to the types of clinical symptoms manifested (Table 3). Cutaneous lesions result from the accumulation of porphyrins in the skin and may result in ulceration and scarring upon exposure to sunlight. Neurological symptoms involve the central nervous system and range from anxiety and

Table 2   Enzyme Deficiencies or Porphyrias

Porphyrin Biosynthesis	Enzyme Deficiency	Porphyria
Glycine + Succinyl−CoA		
ALA Synthetase		
ALA		
ALA Dehydratase		
Porphobilinogen		
Uroporphyrinogen I Synthetase	X	AIP
Uroporphyrinogen III Cosynthetase	X	CEP
Uroporphyrinogen III		
Uroporphyrinogen III Decarboxylase	X	PCT
Coproporphyrinogen III		
Coproporphyrinogen III Oxidase	X	HCP
Protoporphyrinogen IX		
Protoporphyrinogen IX Oxidase	X	VP
Protoporphyrin IX		
Ferrochelatase	X	EP
Heme		

Table 3   Classification of Porphyrias by Clinical Symptoms

CUTANEOUS SYMPTOMS

>   Congenital erythropoietic porphyria (CEP)
>   Erythropoietic protoporphyria (EP)
>   Porphyria cutanea tarda (PCT)

NEUROLOGICAL SYMPTOMS

>   Acute intermittent porphyria (AIP)
>   Variegate porphyria (VP)
>   Hereditary coproporphyria (HCP)

CUTANEOUS AND NEUROLOGICAL SYMPTOMS

>   Variegate porphyria (VP)
>   Hereditary coproporphyria (HCT)

depression to hallucinations, seizures, and coma. Gastrointestinal disturbances usually involve intense abdominal pain, vomiting, and constipation and frequently occur in conjunction with neurological changes.

The porphyrias can also be classified according to the organ in which the biochemical defect occurs—hepatic or erythropoietic (Table 4). In the erythropoietic porphyrias, the enzymatic defect occurs primarily in the bone marrow and an excess quantity of porphyrins accumulates in the normoblasts and erythrocytes.

Three of the hepatic porphyrias (AIP, HCP, VP) are characterized by acute attacks of abdominal pain, tachycardia, and mental and neurological disturbances. Patients with AIP display no cutaneous symptoms whereas approximately 50% of VP patients and 30% of HCP patients can have cutaneous involvement together with the gastrointestinal and neurological

Table 4   Classification of Porphyrias by Organ Involvement

HEPATIC PORPHYRIAS

>   Acute intermittent porphyria (AIP)
>   Variegate porphyria (VP)
>   Hereditary coproporphyria (HCT)
>   Porphyria cutanea tarda (PCT)

ERYTHROPOIETIC PORPHYRIAS

>   Congenital erythropoietic porphyria
>   Erythropoietic protoporphyria

symptoms. All three porphyrias have elevated urine PBG levels during the acute attack but can be distinguished by the fecal porphyrin excretion pattern (see Table 1). The finding of a decreased uroporphyrinogen I synthetase level in red cells identifies AIP.

The remaining hepatic porphyria, PCT, is characterized by the presence of cutaneous photosensitivity and absence of gastrointestinal and neurological symptoms. Excess urine uroporphyrin with normal PBG levels is the most significant biochemical abnormality.

The erythropoietic porphyrias are both characterized by the presence of cutaneous symptoms and the absence of neurological and gastrointestinal symptoms. Both porphyrias develop during childhood and have elevated erythrocyte protoporphyrin levels with normal PBG levels. The urine and fecal porphyrin excretion patterns can aid in the differential diagnosis (see Table 1).

The differential diagnosis of the porphyrias is based on family history, clinical symptoms, porphyrin excretion pattern, and specific enzyme studies. Laboratory tests for porphyrins will vary depending on the type of clinical symptoms. Porphyrias manifesting cutaneous symptoms can be evaluated by analysis of porphyrins in urine, plasma, erythrocytes, or feces. The type of specimen will vary depending on the suspected type of porphyria. Porphyrias manifesting neurological symptoms can be initially evaluated by a screening test for the presence of the porphyrin precursor PBG. A positive test would be followed by a more complete analysis of the porphyrin precursors and porphyrins in urine, plasma, feces, or erythrocytes.

Bibliography

Bissell DM: Laboratory evaluation in porphyria. Semin Liver Dis 2(2):100–107, 1982

Brodie MJ, Goldberg A: Acute hepatic porphyrias. Clin Haematol 9(2):253–272, 1980

Elder GH: The porphyrias: Clinical chemistry, diagnosis and methodology. Clin Haematol 9(2):371–398, 1980

Meyer UA, Schmid R: The porphyrias. In Stanbury JB, Wyngaarden JB, Frederickson DS (eds): The Metabolic Basis of Inherited Disease. New York, McGraw-Hill, 1978

Case 12

A 14-YEAR-OLD BOY sees a local oral surgeon for extraction of two teeth prior to beginning orthodontia. The oral surgeon obtains a weak family history of bleeding. There are four brothers, ages 7 to 17, and a 21-year-old sister in the family. Two of the brothers have a history of prolonged bleeding following dental extractions and of frequent epistaxis (nosebleeds). No other unusual bleeds have been experienced, including none at circumcision of any of the boys.

Because of the bleeding history, the oral surgeon requests a coagulation work-up on the brothers be done prior to performing surgery. The sister is not available for evaluation but by the history given by the mother appears to be normal. The immediate family tree is shown in Figure 3.

What lab procedure(s) would be useful initially as a screen for a possible inherited coagulopathy in this family? (Select as many as appropriate.)

1. Hematocrit and hemoglobin

[
                                                                              ]

2. Platelet count

[
                                                                              ]

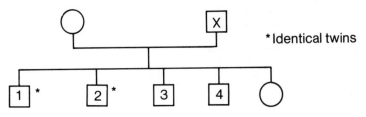

*Identical twins

Figure 3

3. PT, APTT, and TT

4. Kinetic fibrinogen

5. fsp

6. Bleeding time

Section A
What diagnosis is suggested for this family by these lab data? (Select one.)

1. No inherited bleeding disorder is suggested.

Continued

2. Hemophilia A

3. Hemophilia B

4. Type I von Willebrand's disease ("classic")

5. Bernard Soulier disease

Section B

The local laboratory has taken the initial work-up as far as they are able by doing these tests. They now prepare fresh platelet-poor plasma from all four boys, quick-freeze it at −70°C, and ship it on dry ice to a referral coagulation lab. What test(s) would be appropriate to verify the diagnosis of von Willebrand's disease? (Review all choices.)

1. Factor VIII:C

2. Factor VIII:RAg

3. Ristocetin cofactor (VIII:RCo)

Section C

Based on the lab results now available from the referral lab, is the diagnosis of von Willebrand's disease for this family still a possibility? (Select one.)

    1. Unlikely, but still a possibility

    2. Not possible

    3. Is the diagnosis

Section D

The referral lab asks that the brothers come personally to the lab (a distance of 120 miles) so that their evaluation can be continued. What lab procedure(s) should be done at this time? (Choose as many as you feel would be important based on the data obtained to date.)

    1. PT

    2. APTT

3. TT

[   ]

4. Kinetic fibrinogen

[   ]

5. Platelet count

[   ]

6. Bleeding time

[   ]

7. VIII:C

[   ]

8. VIII:RAg

[   ]

Section E

Based on all the clinical and laboratory information you now have, what is the most likely diagnosis for this family? (Select one.)

1. No inherited bleeding disorder is suggested.

[   ]

2. Hemophilia A

[   ]

3. Hemophilia B

[   ]

4. Type I von Willebrand's disease ("classic")

[   ]

5. Bernard Soulier disease

[   ]

Section F

Bleeding time results on all four boys are now normal, whereas this was not true initially. What is the most likely reason for the discrepancy? (Select one.)

1. Diagnosis is von Willebrand's disease, in which there is known to be variability in bleeding time results.

[   ]

2. History of drug ingestion prior to first bleeding time not obtained

[   ]

3. Diagnosis is Bernard Soulier disease.

[   ]

4. Lab error

[   ]

Section G

Brothers 1 and 2 are stated to be identical twins. Based on the results of the lab tests now completed, you can conclude: (Select one.)

1. They are identical twins.

[   ]

2. They may be identical twins.

[   ]

3. They are not identical twins.

[   ]

Section H

Review again the initial lab's APTT results and compare to results the referral lab has now obtained (introductory section, 3, and Section D, 2). Based on this review, what would you say about the initial lab's APTT method? (Select as many as appropriate.)

1. Acceptable method; no reason to consider re-evaluation

[   ]

2. Poor accuracy

[   ]

3. Poor sensitivity

[   ]

Section I

These four brothers have a sister who was unavailable for evaluation at the time of this work-up. Which of the following would be true? (Select one.)

1. The sister may be a carrier of hemophilia B.

2. With three of the four brothers affected, she is *definitely* a carrier of hemophilia B.

3. She cannot be a carrier of hemophilia B because this abnormal gene was a new mutation in this family and thus not carried by the mother.

Enrichment Section

In a male with a history of a mild hemorrhagic disorder and an unclear family history, the differential diagnosis between mild hemophilia and von Willebrand's disease (vWD) may be entertained. Hemophilia A, in particular, may be confused with vWD. The laboratory is instrumental in making the differential diagnosis. The chart on page 122 lists the tests that may be done and that are helpful in differential diagnosis. The results given are those found in clear-cut cases; there are always those mild or borderline cases that give normal or only borderline abnormal results on the screening tests and that need further evaluation. Included, simply because hemophilia B has occurred in this family, are the tests that would identify its presence, although once a decreased level of functional factor IX is verified in a male the diagnosis is clear (assuming there is no acquired cause of factor IX deficiency such as coumarin therapy or liver disease). Because hemophilia A and vWD both result from a defective factor VIII molecule, they can be more easily confused.

Both hemophilia A and B are inherited as a sex-linked recessive disease and thus are expressed primarily in males, although female hemophiliacs have been reported. They have a delay in thrombin generation, and thus in fibrin formation, as their primary manifestation of the disease. Within a family, all affected members can be expected to exhibit the same degree of severity of the disease. Carrier detection is thus of some concern. Women who should be evaluated as possible (but not obligate) carriers include (1) those who have one affected son; (2) those who have an affected

Procedure	Hemophilia A	Type I vWD	Hemophilia B
PT	Normal	Normal	Normal
APTT	Abnormal*	Abnormal*	Abnormal*
TT	Normal	Normal	Normal
Kinetic fibrinogen	Normal	Normal	Normal
Platelet count	Normal	Normal	Normal
Bleeding time	Normal†	Prolonged	Normal†
VIII:C	Decreased	Decreased	Normal
VIII:RAg	Normal to Increased	Decreased	Normal
VIII:RCo	Normal	Decreased	Normal
IX	Normal	Normal	Decreased

* Can be normal, depending on the level of the protein in question and the sensitivity of the procedure used.
† In the absence of drug ingestion (*e.g.,* aspirin, ibuprofen).

brother(s) and/or an affected male relative on the maternal side; and (3) those whose mother is an obligate carrier. Because of lyonization and problems inherent in the tests used, even obligate carriers cannot always be identified by the lab.

Type I von Willebrand's disease is inherited as an autosomal dominant trait with variable penetrance. Thus, expression of the disease in affected family members is variable. In addition, in an affected individual, there is variability over time so that appropriate tests may be randomly abnormal or normal. This can make the diagnosis difficult. It is found with equal frequency in males and females. The primary defect in type I is a decreased synthesis of a normal VIII:RAg (VIII:vWF); this protein is necessary for normal platelet adherence to subendothelial tissue(s). Thus, the primary bleeding manifestations in this syndrome are those of platelet problems (as opposed to procoagulant protein problems such as are seen in hemophilia). Factor VIII:C levels are depressed somewhat equally with VIII:RAg levels; usually these are only mildly decreased. Factor VIII:RCo (ristocetin cofactor) is also equally depressed. This is believed to be a different domain of the same protein as VIII:RAg, and is responsible for agglutination of platelets in the presence of ristocetin.

There are many drugs that affect platelet function; those most commonly found in many over-the-counter medications are aspirin and now the ibuprofen derivatives. Both of these drugs block cyclo-oxygenase, thus preventing the synthesis of thromboxane A_2 (TXA_2) by the platelet (via the prostaglandin pathway). When this is blocked, endogenous release of stored ADP by the platelets is prevented. Since both TXA_2 and ADP are important for normal platelet aggregation, a block in their production and/or release results in delayed platelet aggregation. This gives a prolonged bleeding time in the presence of a normal platelet count, as obtained in this case.

It is important to identify correctly the defect in a patient with an inherited bleeding disorder because the appropriate therapy differs for each. Possible therapeutic regimens and their usefulness in each of the above are listed below:

Regimen	Hemophilia A	vWD	Hemophilia B
Fresh-frozen plasma	Yes	Yes	Yes
Cryoprecipitate	Yes*	Yes*	No
Factor VIII concentrates†	Yes	No	No
Factor IX concentrates†	No	No	Yes

* Preferred.
† Associated with increased hepatitis risk.

Bibliography

Beck WS: Hematology, 3rd ed. Cambridge, MIT Press, 1981

Henry JB: Clinical Diagnosis and Management by Laboratory Methods, 17th ed. Philadelphia, WB Saunders, 1984

Sirridge MS, Shannon R: Laboratory Evaluation of Hemostasis and Thrombosis, 3rd ed. Philadelphia, WB Saunders, 1983

Thompson AR, Harker LA: Manual of Hemostasis and Thrombosis, 3rd ed. Philadelphia, FA Davis, 1983

Williams WJ: Hematology, 3rd ed. New York, McGraw-Hill, 1983

Case 13

A 32-YEAR-OLD WHITE MAN was admitted in the early morning with complaints of acute abdominal pain. The patient was pale and demonstrated malaise and fatigue. He had had a history of frequent headaches and one episode of deep vein thrombosis. The urinalysis showed mild hemoglobinuria. Laboratory data were as follows:

WBC = $3.2 \times 10^3/\mu l$ (4.0–10.0)
RBC = $2.2 \times 10^6/\mu l$ (4.2–5.40)
HGB = 6.1 g/dl (14.0–17.0)
HCT = 19% (42–52)
MCV = 86.4 fl (81–99)
MCH = 26.8 pg (27.0–33.0)
MCHC = 32.1 g/dl (31–35)
PLT = $79 \times 10^3/\mu l$ (150–450)
Differential
    30% neutrophils
    59% lymphocytes
    9% monocytes
    2% eosinophils
Morphology
    Slight polychromatophilia
Bone marrow
    30% cellularity
    M : E ratio = 1 : 1
Coagulation
        PT = 12.5 sec (11–14)
        APTT = 32.0 sec (30–45)

Go to Section A.

Section A
What set of tests would you do in pursuit of a diagnosis? (Select one.)

1. Direct antiglobulin test (DAT)
   Methemalbumin
   Haptoglobin
   Bilirubin
   [   ]

2. Ferritin
   Serum iron
   TIBC
   % Saturation
   [

   ]

3. AST
   ALT
   ALP
   Bilirubin
   Total protein
   Albumin
   Prothrombin time
   [

   ]

4. Serum B_{12}
   Serum folate
   Schilling's test
   Formiminoglutamic acid (FIGLU)
   [

   ]

Section B

DAT (Coombs) = negative
Methemalbumin = present
Haptoglobin = absent
Bilirubin = 2.0 mg/dl

This information suggests which of the following disorders? (Select one.)

1. Hemolytic anemia
   [   ]

2. Iron-deficiency anemia

[   ]

3. Megaloblastic anemia

[   ]

Section C

Which of the following disorders would be the *least* likely to be considered from the available test results under Section B? (Select one.)

1. Sickle cell anemia

[   ]

2. Microangiopathic hemolytic anemia

[   ]

3. AIHA

[   ]

4. Paroxysmal nocturnal hemoglobinuria (PNH)

[   ]

Section D

What one test could be ordered to help separate the hemolytic states in Section C?

1. Sodium metabisulfite

[   ]

2. Peripheral smear

[   ]

3. Ham's test

[   ]

4. Osmotic fragility

[   ]

Section E

The peripheral smear shows a normochromic, normocytic anemia, slight polychromatophilia, and no other morphologic abnormalities. Which of the following hemolytic processes would you continue to pursue? (Select one.)

1. Sickle cell anemia

[   ]

2. Microangiopathic hemolytic anemia

[   ]

3. PNH

[   ]

Section F
What is the basic abnormality in PNH? (Select one.)

1. Defective spectrin—band 4.1 interaction

[   ]

2. Decreased amount of spectrin in the cell wall

[   ]

3. Increased susceptability to the action of complement (C')

[   ]

4. Skeletal instability due to decreased tetramer formation of spectrin

[   ]

Section G
What test would you use to *screen* for PNH? (Select one.)

1. Schumm's test

[   ]

2. Sugar water test

[   ]

3. Osmotic fragility

[   ]

4. Ham's test

[   ]

Section H
What is the mechanism of the sugar water test that causes lysis to be enhanced? (Select one.)

1. Increase in pH

[   ]

2. Lowering the ionic strength of the solution

[   ]

3. Increase in hypotonic solution

[   ]

4. Decreased pH

[   ]

Section I
What disorders can give a false positive sugar water test? (Review all options.)

  1. Leukemias
     [   ]

  2. Myelodysplastic syndromes
     [.   ]

  3. Immune hemolytic anemia
     [   ]

  4. Megaloblastic anemia
     [   ]

Section J
What is the definitive test for PNH? (Select one.)

  1. Schumm's test
     [   ]

  2. Sugar water test
     [   ]

  3. Osmotic fragility
     [   ]

  4. Ham's test
     [   ]

Section K
What is the mechanism that causes lysis to be enhanced in the Ham's test? (Select one.)

  1. Increase in pH
     [   ]

  2. Decrease in pH
     [
                                                                                      ]

  3. Lowering the ionic strength of the solution.
     [   ]

  4. Increase in hypotonic solution
     [   ]

Section L
What constitutes a positive Ham's test in Table 5? (Select one.)

  1. 3+ in tube 2
     1+ in tube 3

Table 5   Procedure for Ham's Test

	Tube 1	Tube 2	Tube 3	Tube 4	Tube 5	Tube 6	Tube 7
Fresh Normal Serum	0.5 ml	0.5 ml			0.5 ml	0.5 ml	
Patient's Serum			0.5 ml				
Heat-Inactivated Normal Serum				0.5 ml			0.5 ml
0.2 N HCl		0.05 ml	0.05 ml	0.05 ml		0.05 ml	0.05 ml
50% Patient's Red Cells	0.05 ml	0.05 ml	0.05 ml	0.05 ml			
50% Normal Red Cells					0.05 ml	0.05 ml	0.05 ml

Other tubes negative
[   ]

2. 3+ in tube 4
   3+ in tube 3
   3+ in tube 2
   [   ]

3. 3+ in tubes 2, 3, 4, 6, and 7
   Other tubes negative
   [   ]

Section M
What two disorders can give a false positive result in tube 2?

1. Hereditary spherocytosis
   [   ]

2. Sideroblastic anemia
   [   ]

3. Iron-deficiency anemia
   [   ]

4. HEMPAS
   [   ]

Section N
Hemolysis due to spherocytosis can occur in tube 2 but also occurs in tube 4 where the cells are suspended in acidified heat-inactivated normal serum. Heat inactivation does not prevent acid hemolysis of spherocytes but it does prevent hemolysis of PNH cells due to inactivation of C'.

Return to Section M and select again or go to Section P.

Section O
In congenital dyserythropoietic anemia (CDA) type II or HEMPAS (hereditary erythroblastic multinuclearity associated with a positive acidified

serum test), the positive test is due to the presence of alloantibodies in normal serum to an unusual antigen present on the CDA type II red cell. Only 30% of the normal population have this particular antibody. It is a naturally occurring IgM antibody that is C' binding. In HEMPAS, lysis does not occur with the patient's own serum (tube 3) and the sugar water test is negative. This helps separate HEMPAS from PNH.

Return to Section M and select again or go to Section P.

Section P
What is the pathogenesis of PNH? (Select one.)
1. Acquired stem cell disorder
   [   ]
2. Hereditary stem cell disorder
   [   ]
3. Renal disease
   [   ]
4. Decreased G-6-PD
   [   ]

Section Q
PNH is an acquired proliferation of a defective stem cell. It appears to be caused by an insult or damage of unknown nature to the bone marrow. These cells are characterized by a membrane that has increased sensitivity to complement. Although this is a clonal disorder, there appear to be two or three red cell populations involved in each patient. These cell types have been separated according to degree of C' sensitivity. PNH-I cells appear normal, have a normal life span, and are Ham's test-negative. PNH-II cells are moderately sensitive to the lytic action of C' (3–5 times normal), have a medium survival, and are Ham's test-positive. PNH-III cells are markedly sensitive to the lytic action of C' (15–25 times normal), have a short survival of about 6 days, and are Ham's test-positive. The majority (>75%) of PNH patients have the combination of type I and type III cells.

Go to Section R.

Section R
What is the biochemical defect in the membrane of a PNH cell? (Select one.)
1. Decreased cholesterol
   [   ]
2. Increased lecithin-to-sphingomyelin ratio
   [   ]

3. Unknown

[

]

4. Decreased ankryin

[   ]

Section S
By what two mechanisms is complement more efficient in lysing PNH red cell membranes?

1. Excess binding of C3 to the membrane

[

]

2. Increased amounts of "membrane attack complexes" (C5–C9)

[   ]

3. Less "membrane attack complexes" (C5–C9) needed for cell lysis

[

]

4. Increased amounts of IgM

[   ]

Section T
What determines the severity of hemolysis in this disorder? (Select one.)

1. The proportion of cells that are type I

[   ]

2. The proportion of cells that are type II

[   ]

3. The proportion of cells that are type III

[

]

Section U
What are some consequences of intravascular hemolysis? (Review all options.)

1. Disseminated intravascular coagulation

[ ]

2. Hemoglobinuria

[ ]

3. Hemosiderinuria

[ ]

4. Iron deficiency

[ ]

5. Acute abdominal or back pain

[ ]

Section V

What may exacerbate a hemolytic crisis in PNH? (Review all options.)

1. Infections

[ ]

2. Surgery

[ ]

3. Transfusions

[ ]

4. Exercise

[ ]

5. Injection of x-ray dyes

[ ]

6. Iron therapy

[ ]

7. Drugs

[   ]

8. Heparin therapy

[   ]

Section W

What is a possible explanation for the low WBC count? (Select one.)

1. Marrow hypoplasia

[

]

2. Antibodies to WBC

[   ]

3. WBC lysis due to C' sensitivity

[

]

4. Infection

[   ]

Section X

What is a possible explanation for the low platelet count? (Select one.)

1. Marrow hypoplasia

[   ]

2. Antibodies to platelets

[   ]

3. Platelet lysis due to C' sensitivity

[

]

4. Bleeding

[   ]

Section Y

What two enzymes are known to be decreased in PNH?

1. LD

[   ]

2. Acetylcholinesterase

[

]

3. Neutrophil alkaline phosphatase (NAP)

[
]

4. Heme synthetase

[   ]

Section Z

What complications are associated with PNH? (Review all options.)

1. Thrombosis

[   ]

2. Marrow aplasia

[
]

3. Renal disease

[
]

4. Infections

[
]

Section AA

Thrombosis is one of the major complications of PNH. By what two mechanisms does this hypercoagulable state occur?

1. Decreased protein C

[   ]

2. Decreased antithrombin III

[   ]

3. Platelet activation by C'

[
]

4. Activation of the clotting system

[
]

Section BB

What type of thrombosis are PNH patients most prone to develop? (Select one.)

1. Arterial thrombosis

   [   ]

2. Venous thrombosis

   [

   ]

3. Ecchymosis

   [   ]

4. Petechiae

   [   ]

Section CC

What treatment is initiated for PNH? (Review all options.)

1. Bone marrow transplant

   [

   ]

2. Transfusions

   [

   ]

3. Iron therapy

   [

   ]

4. Anticoagulants

   [

   ]

5. Hormones

   [

   ]

6. Dextran

   [

   ]

7. Corticosteroids

[   ]

Section DD

What are the possible clinical courses of the disease? (Review all options.)

1. Progresses into aplastic anemia

[   ]

2. Terminates in acute myelogenous leukemia or erythroleukemia

[   ]

3. Evolves into a myeloproliferative disorder

[   ]

4. Evolves into a myelodysplastic disorder

[   ]

5. Death from thrombosis

[   ]

6. Death from infection

[   ]

7. Complete recovery

[   ]

Section EE

Select the clinical finding for which this disease was named. (Select one.)

1. Hematuria at midnight

[   ]

2. Hemoglobin in the urine after sleeping

[   ]

3. Acute lower back pain during sleep

[   ]

Section FF

What is another name for PNH? (Select one.)

1. Ataxia telangiectasia

[   ]

2. Chediak-Higashi syndrome
   [   ]
3. Alder-Reilly anomaly
   [   ]
4. Marchiafava-Micheli syndrome
   [   ]

Enrichment Section

Paroxysmal nocturnal hemoglobinuria is an unusual hemolytic disorder. It normally occurs in persons between the ages of 30 to 50 years, with no sex preference. It is an acquired stem cell disorder where the clonal defect is an abnormal susceptibility of the RBC membrane to the lytic action of complement. The abnormal cells can bind C' more readily. Complement can be activated by either the classical pathway, which requires the presence of antibody, or the alternate pathway, which does not. In this disease it is probably the alternate pathway that is clinically significant. Normally, lysis by the complement system is very inefficient. Several proteins must assemble for the final steps in the lytic pathway. These are C5–C9 and are called the *membrane attack complex.* It takes approximately 25,000 of these complexes per red cell to actually accomplish lysis. It takes only one-tenth the number of these complexes to lyse the very sensitive PNH cells.

There are different populations of red cells ranging from PNH-I, which are normal, to PNH-III, which are very sensitive. The severity of the patient's disease is directly associated with the percentage of PNH-III cells. These may vary from 5% to 95% from patient to patient.

The incidence of this disease is probably much higher, but because of its many forms it is rarely suspected. Often PNH is not diagnosed for 2½ to 3 years from onset of symptoms. PNH should be suspected in a patient with a chronic hemolysis or pancytopenia of unknown origin.

The WBC and platelets are also complement-sensitive although no lysis occurs. Platelets become activated by C' and therefore are strongly implicated as the mechanism for the hypercoagulable state of these patients. The red cell lysis probably also contributes to the activation of the clotting system.

The pancytopenia that exists in many of the patients is due to marrow hypoplasia. The cause is unknown. Therefore, neutropenia is the mechanism that leads to the development of infection and the major cause of death in this disease.

Treatment is basically unsatisfactory. Medical intervention should be kept at a minimum and the patient treated only symptomatically. The survival of these patients averages about 5 years.

Bibliography
Koepke JA: Laboratory Hematology. New York, Churchill Livingstone, 1984
Williams W: Hematology, 3rd ed. New York, McGraw-Hill, 1983
Wintrobe M: Clinical Hematology, 8th ed. Philadelphia, Lea & Febiger, 1981

Case 14

A 65-YEAR-OLD MAN is seen by a physician because of fatigue and frequent nosebleeds. He has also noticed some swelling in the axillary lymph nodes and some reduction in his vision. Laboratory tests reveal the following:

WBC = 4.0 × 10³/μl   (4.0–10.0)
RBC = 4.1 × 10⁶/μl   (4.20–5.40)
HGB = 12.0 g/dl   (14.0–17.0)
HCT = 36%   (42–52)
PLT = 270 × 10³/μl   (150–450)
Total protein = 14.0 g/dl   (6.2–8.2)
Albumin = 2.7 g/dl   (3.5–5.5)

A serum electrophoresis was ordered and it revealed the presence of a monoclonal "spike." What is the incidence of such a spike in the population? (Select one.)

1. A very rare occurrence, <.001%
   [   ]
2. A rare occurrence, <.1%
   [   ]
3. Not a rare occurrence, >.1%
   [

   ]

Section A
The next step in the laboratory work-up is to characterize the monoclonal protein. Which of the following tests could be used to characterize the monoclonal immunoglobulin? (Select as many as appropriate.)

1. Serum immunoelectrophoresis

[
]

2. Urine immunoelectrophoresis

[
]

3. Quantitation of serum immunoglobulins

[
]

4. Quantitation of urine proteinuria

[
]

Section B

Based on the incidence of occurrence, select the most common and the least common immunoglobulin types found in association with an electrophoretic spike.

1. IgA

[   ]

2. IgD

[   ]

3. IgE

[
]

4. IgG

[
]

5. IgM

[   ]

Section C

The serum immunoelectrophoresis identified the immunoglobulin as IgM with kappa (k) chains. From the following list of diseases, select those that can be associated with increased levels of IgM. (Review each option.)

1. Multiple myeloma

[
]

2. Benign monoclonalgammopathy (BMG)

[   ]

3. Waldenström's macroglobulinemia

[   ]

4. Lymphoma

[   ]

Section D
Multiple myeloma is a malignant neoplasm of a single clone of plasma cells of the bone marrow. Choose the typical characteristics of multiple myeloma. (Select as many as appropriate.)

1. Occurs in persons under 40 years of age

[   ]

2. Occurs in persons over 40 years of age

[   ]

3. There is a higher incidence in males.

[   ]

4. There is a higher incidence in females.

[   ]

5. Bone pain

[   ]

6. No bone pain

[   ]

7. Bone destruction

[   ]

8. No bone destruction

[   ]

9. Renal abnormalities

[   ]

10. No renal abnormalities

[ ]

Section E
Select the typical blood findings in multiple myeloma. (Select as many as appropriate.)

1. Microcytic, hypochromic anemia

[ ]

2. Macrocytic anemia

[ ]

3. Normocytic, normochromic anemia

[ ]

4. Decreased WBC

[ ]

5. Normal platelet count

[ ]

Section F
Select the bone marrow findings that are common in multiple myeloma. (Select one.)

1. Normal numbers of normal plasma cells

[ ]

2. Increased numbers of normal plasma cells

[ ]

3. Increased numbers of abnormal plasma cells

[ ]

Section G
Bone lesions and bone pain are the most common symptoms in multiple myeloma. Select the laboratory findings that are associated with these symptoms. (Select as many as appropriate.)

1. Serum calcium decreased
   [   ]

2. Serum calcium increased
   [

   ]

3. Serum alkaline phosphatase decreased
   [   ]

4. Serum alkaline phosphatase normal
   [

   ]

5. Serum alkaline phosphatase increased
   [   ]

6. Serum phosphorus decreased
   [   ]

7. Serum phosphorus normal
   [

   ]

Section H

BMG is often discovered only incidentally during the diagnosis of an unrelated illness. It is characterized by the presence of a homogeneous immunoglobulin in the urine or plasma, or in both. From the following,
select the parameters that favor the diagnosis of BMG. (Select as many as
appropriate.)

1. Serum IgG concentrations of <2.0 g/dl
   [

   ]

2. Serum IgA or IgM concentrations of <2.0 g/dl
   [   ]

3. Serum IgA or IgM concentrations of <1.0 g/dl
   [

   ]

4. Serum IgD or IgE concentrations of <1.0 g/dl
   [   ]

5. The absence of IgD or IgE paraproteins
   [

   ]

6. A progressive spike

[   ]

7. A nonprogressive or transient spike

[
                                                    ]

8. Decreased serum concentrations of the other immunoglobulins

[   ]

9. Normal serum concentrations of the other immunoglobulins

[
                                                    ]

10. Absence of Bence Jones protein

[
                                                    ]

11. Presence of Bence Jones protein

[   ]

12. Decreased serum albumin

[   ]

13. Normal serum albumin

[
                                                    ]

14. Skeletal lesions

[   ]

15. No skeletal lesions

[
                                                    ]

16. Bone marrow plasmacytosis of >10% or an increase in lymphocytes

[   ]

17. Bone marrow plasmacytosis of >10% and no increase in lymphocytes

[
                                                    ]

Section I

Malignant lymphoma is a neoplastic proliferation of one of the cell types of the lymphopoietic–reticular tissue. Usually lymphoma begins in and involves predominantly lymph nodes, although other sites may be involved. About 20% of the patients with lymphoma produce paraproteins that are usually of the IgM type.

Go to Section K.

Section J

Waldenström's macroglobulinemia appears to be a variant of chronic lymphocytic leukemia or well-differentiated lymphocytic lymphoma. The paraprotein is invariably IgM and is produced by the most mature B-lymphocytes. Select the clinical features that are associated with Waldenström's macroglobulinemia. (Select as many as appropriate.)

1. The average age at manifestation is <50 years.

    [   ]

2. The average age at manifestation is >50 years.

3. There is a higher incidence in males.

4. There is a higher incidence in females.

    [   ]

5. Normal lymph nodes, liver, and spleen

    [   ]

6. Enlarged lymph nodes, liver, and spleen

7. A bleeding diathesis

8. No bleeding diathesis

    [   ]

9. Presence of osteolytic bone lesions

10. Absence of osteolytic bone lesions

11. Ocular changes

Continued

12. Presence of bone pain

13. Absence of bone pain

14. Neurological disturbances

Section K

Urine electrophoresis was performed on this patient and Bence Jones protein was present. Bence Jones proteinuria is found in approximately one-third of the patients with macroglobulinemia. Renal pathology has been associated with the presence of Bence Jones proteinuria. Although renal disease is much less common than in multiple myeloma, select the mechanism that produces the renal abnormalities. (Select as many as appropriate.)

1. Occlusion of tubules by casts

2. Amyloid deposits in the kidney

3. Interstitial infiltration by malignant cells

4. Occlusion of glomerulus by deposits of IgM proteins

Section L

Most of the clinical manifestations are related to the properties of the macroglobulins. Most patients experience "hyperviscosity syndrome." The viscosity of the blood is influenced by the molecular size and shape of the macroglobulin as well as its tendency to aggregate. Select the clinical manifestations related to the hyperviscosity. (Select as many as appropriate.)

1. Distended retinal veins and retinal hemorrhages

[   ]

2. Impaired kidney function

[   ]

3. Congestive heart failure

[   ]

4. Decreased capillary circulation in the extremities

[   ]

Section M

Anemia is the most common presenting feature of macroglobulinemia. In most instances the anemia is normochromic, normocytic. Select the mechanisms involved in producing the anemia. (Select as many as appropriate).

1. Inadequate red cell production

[   ]

2. Hemolysis

[   ]

3. Shortened red cell survival

[   ]

4. Blood loss

[   ]

Section N

What would be the expected WBC? (Select one.)

1. Increased

[   ]

2. Normal

[   ]

3. Decreased

[
                                                                    ]

Section O

What would be the expected erythrocyte sedimentation rate? (Select one.)

1. Increased

[
                                                                    ]

2. Normal

[   ]

Section P

Patients with macroglobulinemia present with bruising, purpura, epistaxis, and bleeding from mucosal surfaces. What would be expected in regard to the platelets? (Select two.)

1. Decreased platelet count

[   ]

2. Normal platelet count

[   ]

3. Impaired platelet function

[   ]

4. Normal platelet function

[   ]

Section Q

Which of the following tests would be abnormal in macroglobulinemia? (Select as many as appropriate.)

1. Bleeding time

[   ]

2. Tourniquet test

[   ]

3. Clot retraction

[   ]

4. Prothrombin time (PT)

[   ]

5. Activated partial thromboplastin time (APTT)

[   ]

6. Prothrombin consumption (PTC)

[   ]

7. Thrombin time

[   ]

8. Platelet aggregation

[

]

Section R

Some IgM proteins may interact with labile coagulation factors to inhibit coagulation, which is usually detected by a prolonged PT. It is unclear if the paraprotein coats the intact fibrinogen molecule or fibrin monomer after generation from fibrinogen. It is proposed that the F(ab) sites on the immunoglobulin bind to fibrin during the clotting process. This inhibits fibrin monomer aggregation.

Go back to Section Q and select again or go to Section T.

Section S

Inhibitors of coagulation factors have been reported. These include inhibitors of factor VIII, prothrombin complex, V, VII, and X. Reduced levels of factors II, V, VII, X, and XI have also been described. Bleeding diathesis may result with the formation of complexes between macroglobulins and specific clotting factors such as factor VIII.

Go back to Section Q and select again or go to Section T.

Section T

Often, the bone marrow cannot be aspirated because of the great cellularity of the marrow combined with the increased viscosity of the tissue fluid. But if marrow is sampled, what are the typical features found in the bone marrow? (Select as many as appropriate.)

1. Increased erythroid precursors

[   ]

2. Increased myeloid precursors

[   ]

3. Increased lymphoid cells

[

]

4. Decreased eosinophils

[   ]

5. Increased eosinophils

[   ]

6. Decreased basophils and mast cells
[   ]

7. Increased basophils and mast cells

[   ]

8. Periodic acid–Schiff (PAS)-stain negative
[   ]

9. PAS-stain positive

[   ]

Section U

For each of the following laboratory determinations, select the characteristic finding associated with macroglobulinemia. (Select one for each determination.)

Total Serum Protein

1. Decreased
[   ]

2. Normal
[   ]

3. Increased
[   ]

Serum Albumin

1. Decreased
[   ]

2. Normal
[   ]

3. Increased
[   ]

A/G Ratio

1. Normal
[   ]

2. Inverted
   [   ]

Serum Calcium

1. Decreased
   [   ]
2. Normal
   [   ]
3. Increased
   [   ]

Serum Phosphorus

1. Decreased
   [   ]
2. Normal
   [   ]
3. Increased
   [   ]

Serum Alkaline Phosphatase

1. Decreased
   [   ]
2. Normal
   [   ]
3. Increased
   [   ]

Blood Urea Nitrogen

1. Decreased
   [   ]
2. Normal
   [   ]
3. Increased
   [   ]

Serum Creatinine

1. Decreased
   [   ]
2. Normal
   [   ]

3. Increased
[   ]

Lactic Dehydrogenase (LD)

1. Decreased
[   ]

2. Normal
[   ]

3. Increased
[   ]

Total Bilirubin

1. Decreased
[   ]

2. Normal
[   ]

3. Increased
[   ]

Serum Uric Acid

1. Decreased
[   ]

2. Normal
[   ]

3. Increased
[
                                                                        ]

IgG Levels

1. Decreased
[   ]

2. Normal
[   ]

3. Increased
[   ]

IgM Levels

1. Decreased
[   ]

2. Normal
[   ]

3. Increased
[   ]

IgA Levels

1. Decreased
[   ]

2. Normal
[   ]

3. Increased
[   ]

Haptoglobin Levels

1. Decreased

[   ]

2. Normal
[   ]

3. Increased
[   ]

C3 Levels

1. Decreased

[   ]

2. Normal
[   ]

3. Increased
[   ]

C4 Levels

1. Decreased
[   ]

2. Normal
[   ]

3. Increased
[   ]

Alpha₁-Acid Glycoprotein Levels

1. Decreased
[   ]

2. Normal

[   ]

3. Increased

[   ]

Alpha₁-Antitrypsin Levels

1. Decreased

[   ]

2. Normal

[   ]

3. Increased

[   ]

Transferrin Levels

1. Decreased

[   ]

2. Normal

[   ]

3. Increased

[   ]

Cold Agglutinins

1. Negative

[   ]

2. Positive

[   ]

Cryoglobulins

1. Negative

[   ]

2. Positive

[   ]

Bence Jones Protein

1. Negative

[   ]

2. Positive

[

]

Serum Sodium

1. Decreased

[   ]

2. Normal

[   ]

3. Increased

[   ]

Serum Potassium

1. Decreased

[   ]

2. Normal

[   ]

3. Increased

[   ]

Serum Chloride

1. Decreased

[   ]

2. Normal

[   ]

3. Increased

[   ]

Serum Bicarbonate

1. Decreased

[   ]

2. Normal

[   ]

3. Increased

[   ]

Anion Gap

1. Decreased

[   ]

2. Normal

[   ]

3. Increased

[   ]

Serum Cholesterol

1. Decreased

[   ]

2. Normal

[   ]

3. Increased

[   ]

Relative Serum Viscosity

1. Decreased

[   ]

2. Normal

[   ]

3. Increased

[   ]

Sia Water Test

1. Negative

[   ]

2. Positive

[   ]

Section V

The anion gap can be calculated from the following formula:

$$\text{Anion gap} = Na^+ + K^+ - (Cl^- + HCO_3^-)$$

The low anion gap is due to the retention of Cl^- and HCO_3^- to offset the cationic charge of the monoclonal immunoglobulins.

Go back to Section U.

Section W
Go back to the introduction and read the case history and the laboratory data. In light of these data, select the most probable diagnosis. (Select one.)

1. Multiple myeloma
   [   ]
2. BMG
   [   ]
3. Waldenström's macroglobulinemia
   [   ]
4. Lymphoma
   [   ]

Enrichment Section
Waldenström's macroglobulinemia was described in 1944 as a neoplasm arising from the plasma cell and lymphoid cell populations that are normally responsible for the synthesis of immunoglobulins containing μ heavy chains. The immature B-lymphocytes seem to be the cells affected and they secrete the monoclonal IgM. Proliferation of the abnormal lymphocytoid cells leads to enlargement of the spleen and lymph nodes and there may be an infiltration of the liver, kidneys, and other viscera. The clinical manifestations are related to the properties of the macroglobulins. There may be neurological manifestations, ranging from headaches, dizziness, and vertigo, to somnolence, stupor, and coma. Other symptoms include weakness, fatigue, and anorexia. Hematological complications include bleeding manifestations, which may be aggravated by the effects of the macroglobulins on the clotting system.

The diagnosis of Waldenström's macroglobulinemia is confirmed by electrophoresis that reveals a homogeneous spike in the beta to gamma region, and by immunoelectrophoresis that confirms the IgM nature of the spike.

Treatment for Waldenström's macroglobulinemia consists of steroids, chlorambucil, cyclophosphamide, and other chemotherapeutic agents used in different combinations. Plasmapheresis is used to reduce the serum IgM concentration and thus hyperviscosity and cryoglobulinemia.

The median survival period is about 50 months in those patients who respond to chemotherapy and about 24 months in those who don't respond. Death is generally due to severe anemia, hemorrhage, or infections. However, infections are less common in macroglobulinemia than in multiple myeloma.

Bibliography
Beck WS: Hematology, 4th ed. Cambridge, MIT Press, 1985
Brown SS, Mitchell FL, Young DS: Chemical Diagnosis of Disease. Amsterdam, Elsevier/North-Holland Biomedical Press, 1979
Deuel TF, Davis P: Waldenström's macroglobulinemia. Arch Intern Med 143:986–988, 1983
Henry JB: Clinical Diagnosis and Management by Laboratory Methods, 17th ed. Philadelphia, WB Saunders, 1984
Tietz NW: Textbook of Clinical Chemistry. Philadelphia, WB Saunders, 1985
Williams WJ: Hematology, 3rd ed. New York, McGraw-Hill, 1983
Wintrobe MW: Clinical Hematology, 8th ed. Philadelphia, Lea & Febiger, 1981

Case 15

A 41-YEAR-OLD WOMAN is referred for a coagulation work-up because of "hypercoagulable state." She began having thrombotic problems when she was in her early twenties. At that time, over a period of 5 years, she underwent surgery four times: hemorrhoidectomy, hysterectomy, appendectomy, and cholecystectomy. All these procedures were considered necessary because of thrombotic obstruction. Since these surgeries, she has had a general history of angina, hypertension, and thrombosis, including numerous episodes of deep venous thrombosis (DVT), superficial venous thrombosis (SVT), and pulmonary emboli. Both of her parents had a history of cardiovascular illness, both dying of strokes (mother at age 56, father at 65). She has been treated in the past with coumarin therapy; however, compliance in taking the drug has been questioned.

She is admitted to the hospital for her coagulation work-up. (Select as many of the following test(s) as you feel would be appropriate as part of her initial screening.)

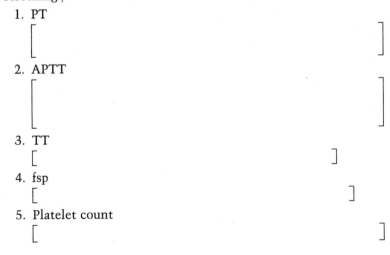

1. PT
   [   ]

2. APTT
   [   ]

3. TT
   [   ]

4. fsp
   [   ]

5. Platelet count
   [   ]

6. Bleeding time

[   ]

7. Kinetic fibrinogen

[   ]

8. Antithrombin III (AT III)

[   ]

9. Hematocrit and hemoglobin

[   ]

Section A

Based on the coagulation data obtained and her clinical history, you can conclude which of the following to be true?

1. Patient has a normal hemostatic system; no cause of her thromboses can be identified.

[

]

2. Further test(s) need to be done to attempt to identify the etiology for her thrombotic episodes.

[

]

3. Patient has a normal AT III at a time of a thrombotic episode; therefore, AT III deficiency may be the etiology of her thrombotic disease.

[

]

4. Patient has a mild iron deficiency due to chronic blood loss so this is evidence of a hemorrhagic tendency and further work-up should be done.

[

]

[   ]

Section B

Before continuing in the evaluation of this patient, it is important to consider general possible causes of thrombosis in *any* patient. (Select as many
of these as you feel are potential causes.)

1. Deficient or abnormal AT III
[   ]

2. Deficient or abnormal plasminogen
[   ]

3. Deficiency in antiplasmin
[   ]

4. Deficient or abnormal tissue plasminogen activator (tPA)
[   ]

5. Defective release of tissue plasminogen activator (tPA)
[   ]

6. Deficient or abnormal protein C
[   ]

7. Deficiency in factor VIII : C
[   ]

8. Abnormal fibrinogen (dysfibrinogen)
[   ]

Section C

The following procedures are done next in an attempt to identify the
etiology of this woman's thromboses.

	Result	Reference Range
Factor V	175%	50%–150%
Factor VIII : C	535%	50%–200%
Euglobulin clot lysis time (ELT)	9.4 hr	2–4 hr

Based on the information known to this point, select any of the following that may be the etiology of her thrombotic problems.

1. AT III deficiency

[

]

2. Defective AT III

[

]

3. Increased concentration of factors V and VIII : C

[

]

4. Defective plasminogen

[

]

5. Deficiency of plasminogen

[

]

6. Defective activation of plasminogen

[

]

Section D

Since factors V and VIII : C are increased, it is important to consider them as at least part of the etiology. The most likely reason for these to be increased to these levels in *this* patient is which of the following? (Select one.)

1. These are both acute phase proteins and are simply elevated in this patient as part of the inflammatory response.

[

]

2. There is a deficiency of protein C.

[

]

3. There is a defect in the fibrinolytic system.

[

]

Section E

Protein C levels are measured, and a normal value is obtained. Given this information, the next most appropriate area to consider would be which of the following?

1. V and VIII : C are both acute phase proteins and are simply elevated in this patient as part of the inflammatory response.

[   ]

2. There is a defect in the fibrinolytic system.

[

]

Section F

In evaluating the fibrinolytic system, a euglobulin clot lysis time (ELT) has already been performed and a result of 9.4 hours (reference range 2–4 hours) obtained. The ELT is initially done by precipitating the euglobulin fraction from the patient's plasma. This contains plasminogen, plasminogen activator (tissue plasminogen activator [tPA]), and fibrinogen, but it does not contain any inhibitors of the fibrinolytic system. After isolating this fraction, it is then redissolved, allowed to clot, and the clot incubated at 37°C and observed over time for lysis. (Select as many of the following that may contribute to this abnormal clot lysis.)

1. Deficient plasminogen

[

]

2. Abnormal plasminogen

[

]

3. Deficient tissue plasminogen activator (tPA)

[

]

4. Abnormal tissue plasminogen activator (tPA)

$$\left[\right]$$

Section G

The ELT is now repeated, with additions made to the initial system in an attempt to separate possible causes of the abnormal lysis time. The following results are obtained:

	Result	Reference Range
ELT with normal plasminogen added	8.2 hr	2–4 hr
ELT with streptokinase added	3 hr	
ELT with urokinase added	2.5 hr	

Given these results, the etiology for this patient's thrombotic disease now appears to be: (Select as many as appropriate.)

1. An abnormal plasminogen

$$\left[\right]$$

2. A deficiency of tissue plasminogen activator (tPA)

$$\left[\right]$$

3. An abnormal tissue plasminogen activator (tPA)

$$\left[\right]$$

Enrichment Section

Thrombotic disease, along with its complications, is a major medical concern, particularly in the Western World where it plays a major role in both morbidity and mortality. Until recently, tests were not available to aid in the evaluation of patients who presented with multiple thrombotic episodes or of families with an affected member. With increased understanding, there now are available a number of procedures to help identify the etiology of disease in these patients.

Probably the first protein deficiency to be associated with an increased risk of thrombosis was that of antithrombin III (AT III). Later, once an immunologic assay became available for AT III it was demonstrated that there are rare families who seem to have an abnormal AT III (as opposed to a deficiency). AT III is an alpha-2 globulin that inhibits serine proteases (XIIa, XIa, IXa, Xa, and IIa [thrombin]). *In vitro*, in the absence of heparin, it only slowly inhibits these proteases; however, in the presence of heparin, it rapidly inhibits them. *In vivo*, AT III apparently interacts with the damaged endothelial cell surface ("heparinoid substance"), and is then an immediate potent inhibitor of these proteases.

The lupus anticoagulant (lupus inhibitor) is an acquired immunoglobulin inhibitor that prolongs phospholipid-dependent tests, particularly the APTT. It was first described in patients with systemic lupus erythematosus (SLE), hence the name, but it is not exclusive to SLE and is found in other patients. Interestingly, although it behaves like an anticoagulant *in vitro*, prolonging some tests, patients with the lupus anticoagulant do not have prolonged bleeding. In fact, 25% to 50% of them will develop at least one thrombotic episode, and many have recurrent thromboses.

Protein C is a vitamin K-dependent protein, which, when activated, destroys activated factors Va and VIIIa, thus acting as a major control of the clotting process. As thrombin is generated and released into the circulation, it binds to a receptor found on the surface of the endothelial cells, thrombomodulin. This complex (thrombin–thrombomodulin) activates protein C; protein S is required as a co-factor. In the absence of activated protein C, factor V and factor VIII levels increase, and these have been associated with a higher risk of thrombosis.

The fibrinolytic system is instrumental in controlled lysis of a clot once formed. There are various activators of plasminogen, the most important of which, physiologically, appears to be that released by damaged endothelial cells, known as tissue plasminogen activator (tPA). tPA is only activated in the presence of fibrin; thus, it requires the presence of a clot before it can activate plasminogen. Defects in this system again have been associated with a higher incidence of thrombosis.

Patients with a deficiency of plasminogen understandably have delayed removal of clots. With the availability of immunologic assays for plasminogen, patients have been identified who have a defective plasminogen protein, one that cannot be appropriately activated by tissue plasminogen activator (tPA) or by urokinase (UK) but that can often be activated by streptokinase (SK). Since SK is the primary activator of plasminogen used in *in vitro* tests measuring plasminogen (although it is not a physiological activator and its mechanism of activation of plasminogen differs from that of tPA and UK), normal results may be obtained. However, in these patients, when UK is used as the activator in these same tests, abnormal results are often obtained.

In the euglobulin clot lysis time (ELT), tissue plasminogen activator from the patient is the activator of plasminogen. If it is deficient or abnormal, prolonged clot lysis times will occur. The patient in this case study appears to have either a deficiency of tPA or an abnormal tPA because the results became normal when the patient's plasminogen was activated with both SK and UK. These two could be separated, at least theoretically, by an immunologic assay for tPA; an abnormality would show evidence of the protein being present whereas a deficiency would not. If it is a deficiency, the etiology is unknown; it could be due to a true deficiency in synthesis of the protein, *or* it could be a result of defective release of tPA by endothelial cells into plasma. At this point in time, there are very few labs that can separate out these possibilities.

The evaluation of patients with hypercoagulable states is in its infancy but is growing at a rapid rate as more is learned and understood about thrombosis. This means more tests are being developed and/or proposed to aid in diagnosis. Hopefully, as identification of the etiology of thrombosis in a patient improves, therapeutic intervention will become more effective and the consequences of thrombotic disease will diminish.

Bibliography

Beck WS: Hematology, 3rd ed. Cambridge, MIT Press, 1981

Henry JB: Clinical Diagnosis and Management by Laboratory Methods, 17th ed. Philadelphia, WB Saunders, 1984

Sirridge MS, Shannon R: Laboratory Evaluation of Hemostasis and Thrombosis, 3rd ed. Philadelphia, WB Saunders, 1983

Thompson AR, Harker LA: Manual of Hemostasis and Thrombosis, 3rd ed. Philadelphia, FA Davis, 1983

Williams WJ: Hematology, 3rd ed. New York, McGraw-Hill, 1983